Blood Pressure Control

a matter of choices

by

Nancy R. Hull, B.A.
W. Dallas Hall, M.D.
Julia Ann Purcell, R.N., M.N., CCRN
Yvonne Payne, R.D., L.D.

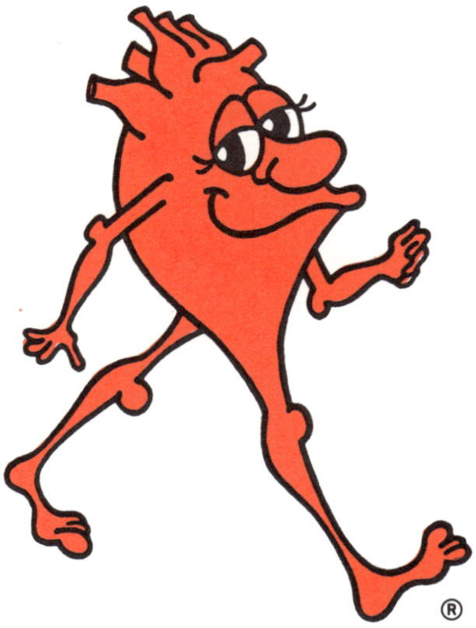

This book is written to help you find out more about hypertension. It should not be used to replace any of your doctor's advice or treatment.

More about the authors:

Nancy R. Hull, B.A., serves as an editor and art director for Pritchett & Hull Associates, Inc., a company she co-owns.

W. Dallas Hall, M.D., is Professor of Medicine and Director of The Division of Hypertension at Emory University School of Medicine and Grady Memorial Hospital, Atlanta, GA.

Julia Ann Purcell, R.N., M.N., CCRN, is a Clinical Nursing Specialist in Cardiology at Emory University Hospital, Atlanta, GA. She has authored many patient publications in the area of heart disease.

Yvonne Payne, R.D., L.D., is a registered and licensed dietitian specializing in cardiac nutrition in the Cardiac Clinic at Grady Memorial Hospital, Atlanta, GA. She has written numerous articles on nutrition and is a member of the Nutrition Committee of the American Heart Association, Georgia Affiliate.

Reviewer:
Janet Cope, M.P.H., Atlanta, GA, has been involved for many years in the area of public health nutrition.

Design, Illustrations: **Michele Williams, Nancy Hull**
Editing: **Faye Hoffman**
Pritchett & Hull Associates, Inc., Atlanta, GA

A matter of choices

Control of high blood pressure (also called "hypertension") is a matter of choices. Your doctor can call the plays, but you will have to carry the ball. Pills can't do it all for you. You must perform the magic and choose the health habits that keep your blood pressure within a normal range for you.

In the early stages, hypertension causes few problems. Most people are not even aware that they have it. But over the years, uncontrolled high blood pressure begins to damage the heart, blood vessels, brain, eyes and kidneys. Without treatment, the risks for heart failure, heart attack, stroke, kidney failure or reduced eyesight are great.

You can help prevent these risks by making wise choices about foods, exercise, medications and stress. Ask questions when you have them. Talk with your doctor if you think some part of your treatment is not working. The choices you make will be the key to how well you control high blood pressure and your health.

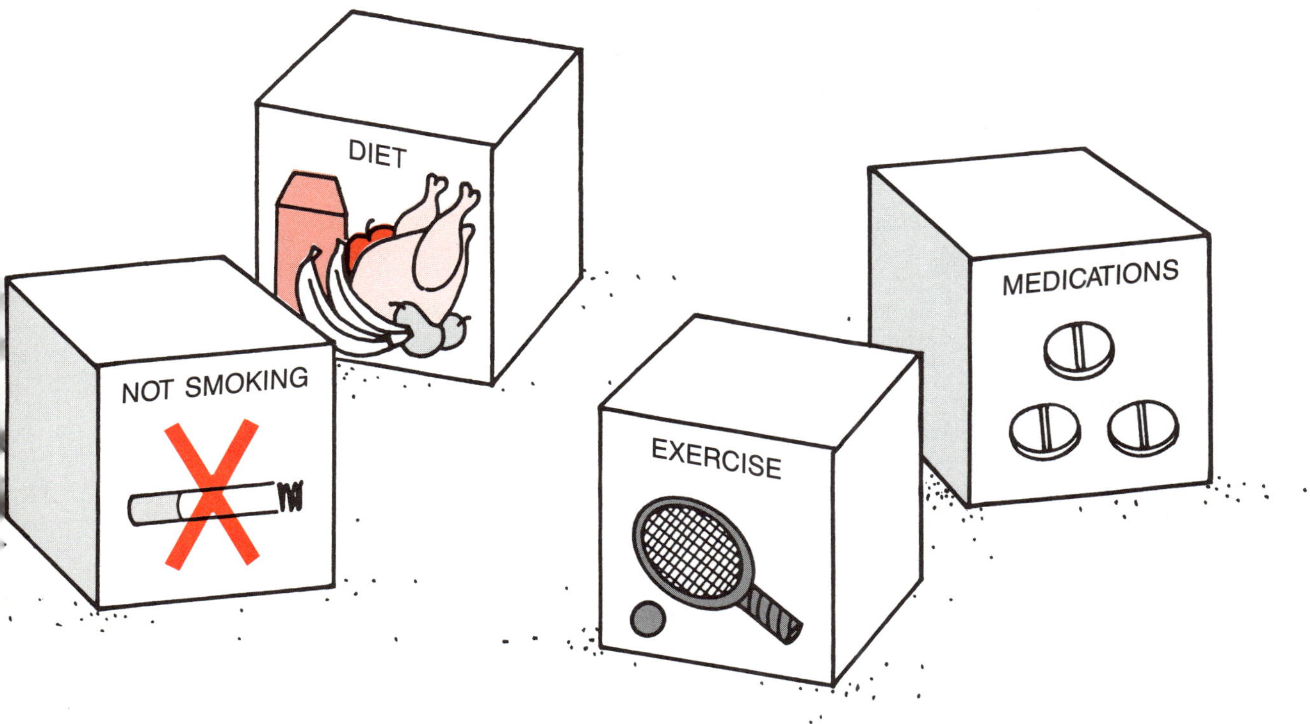

Table of contents

Start making choices right now. Read this book in any order that suits you.

A matter of choices 3

Blood pressure 6-11
- **When blood pressure is normal** 6-7
- **When blood pressure is high** 8
- **Types of high blood pressure** 9
- **People with hypertension** 10-11

Treatment 12-41
- **What you eat** 13-31
  - Sodium 14
  - How to fix low-sodium foods 15
  - Low-sodium foods—what to buy 16-17
  - High-sodium foods—AVOID 18-19
  - Fats and cholesterol 20
  - How to fix low-fat, low-cholesterol foods 21
  - Low-fat, low-cholesterol foods—what to buy 22-23
  - High-fat, high-cholesterol foods—AVOID 24-25
  - Potassium 26
  - High-potassium foods—what to buy 27
  - Balanced meals 28
  - Food labels 29
  - Mystery foods 30
  - Alcohol 30
  - Snacks 31
- **Body weight** 32-33
- **Medications** 34-35
- **Relaxation** 36-37
- **Regular exercise** 38-40
- **Not smoking** 41

Taking your own blood pressure 42-47
Types of equipment 43-44
Technique 45-47

Some final words 48

Resources . . . . inside back cover

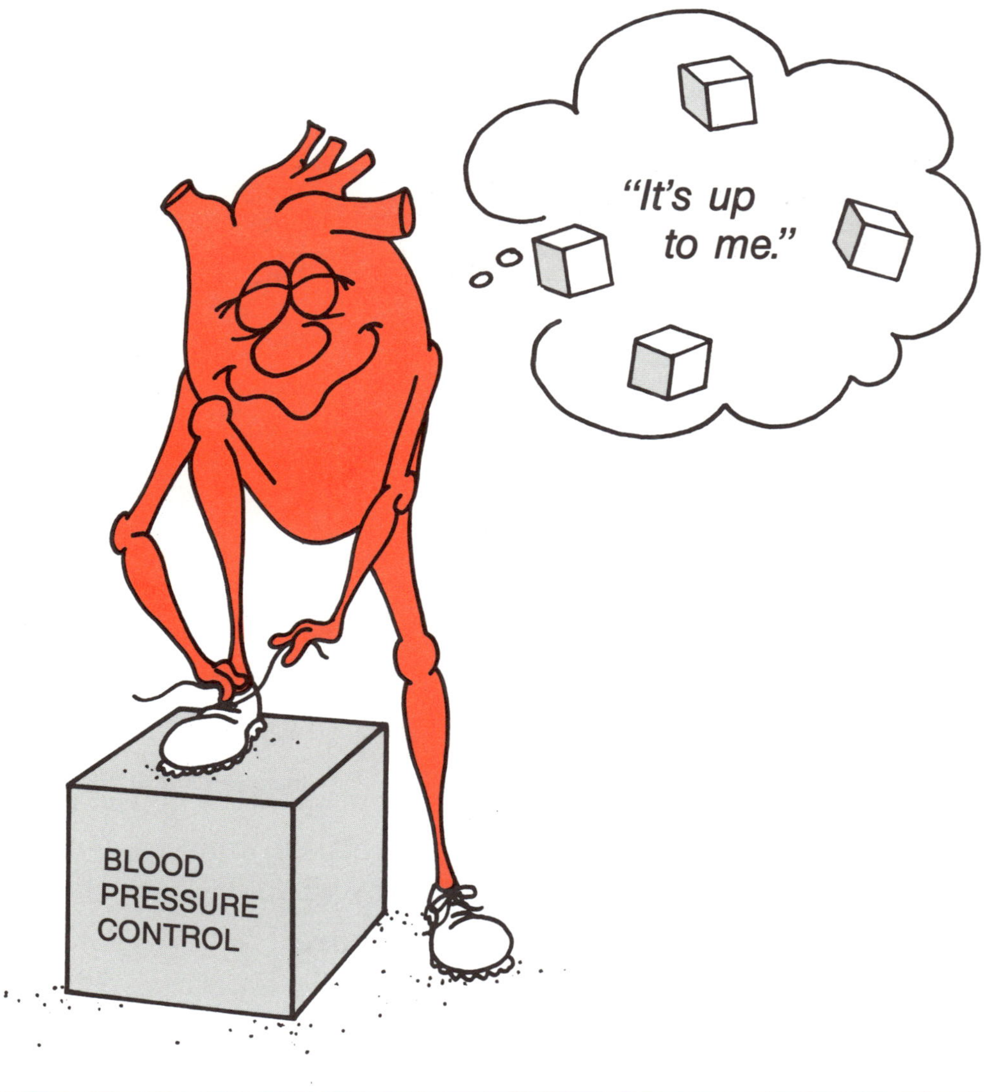

Blood pressure

When blood pressure is normal

Blood pressure (BP) is the force that moving blood puts on the artery walls. As the heart muscle pumps out blood, the aorta (main blood vessel) is stretched until a peak pressure is reached. This peak pressure is called the **"systolic pressure."** It is normal for the systolic pressure to go up for a time during exercise or stress.

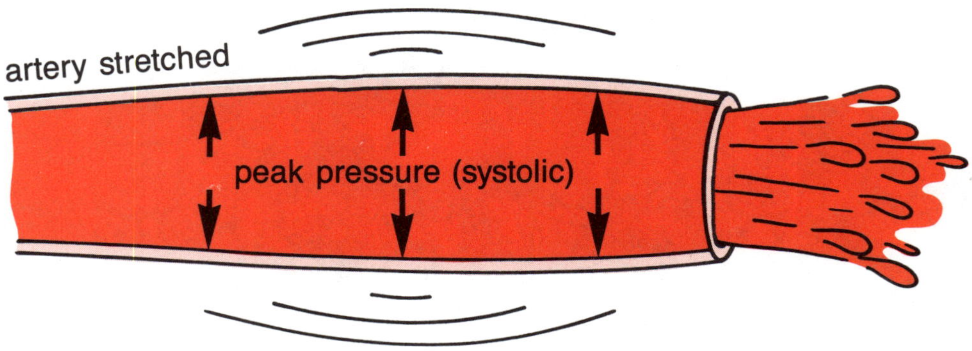

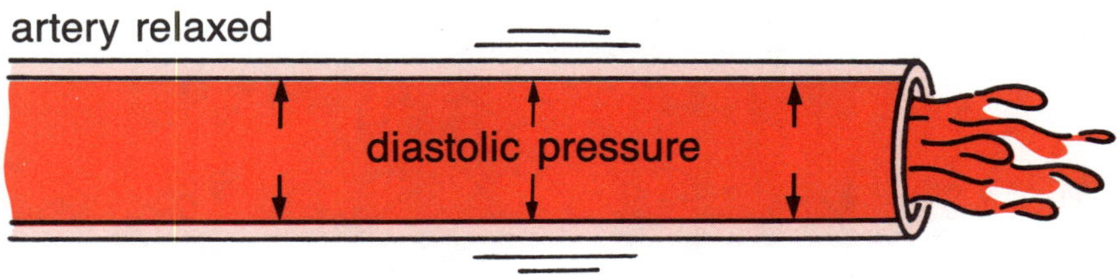

Between heartbeats, the arteries are more relaxed, but they stay tense enough for smooth blood flow to all parts of the body. This tension is the **"diastolic pressure."** The diastolic pressure should stay the same or be a little lower during exercise such as walking, jogging or dancing.

Systolic pressure

Peak pressure in arteries when heart pumps out the blood to the body.

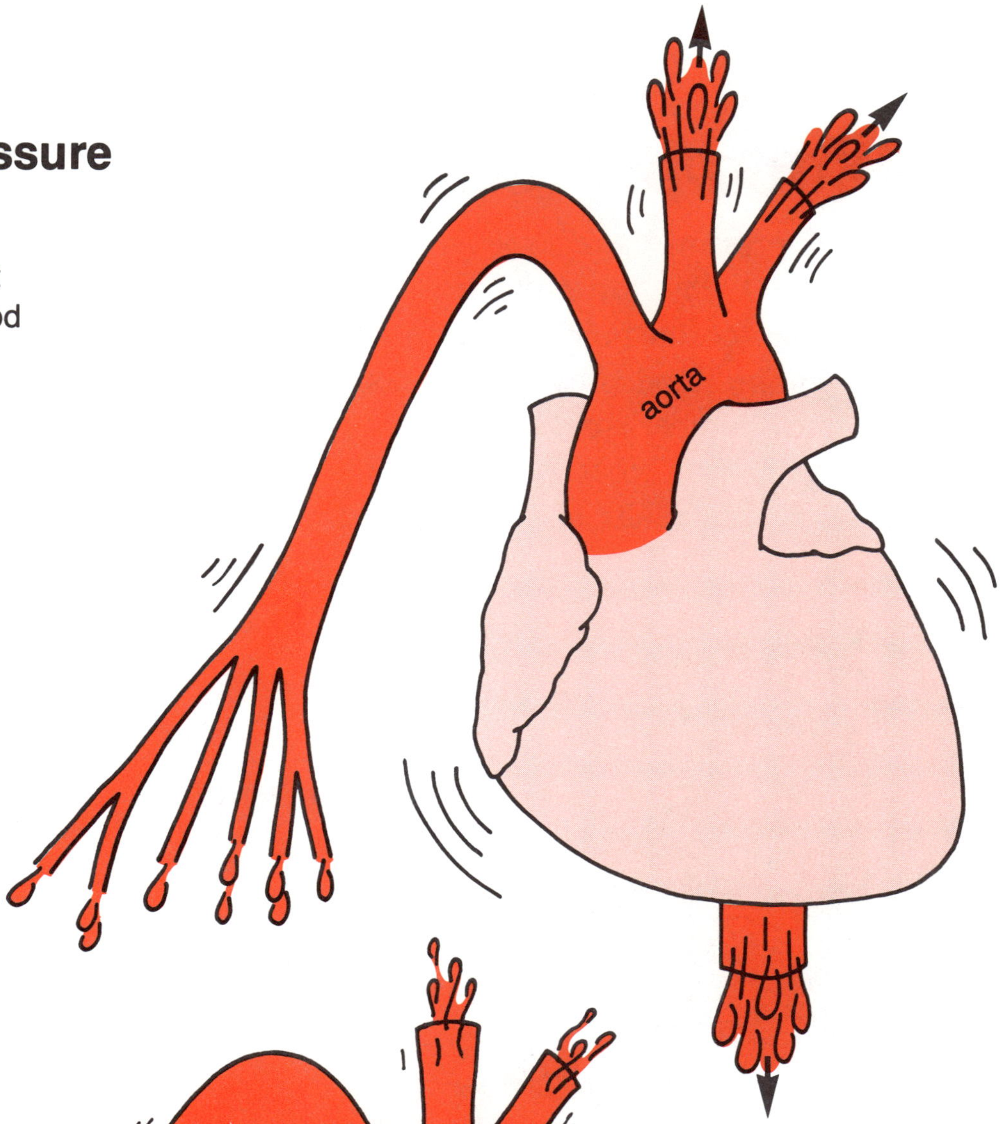

Diastolic pressure

Pressure left in arteries after heart has pumped.

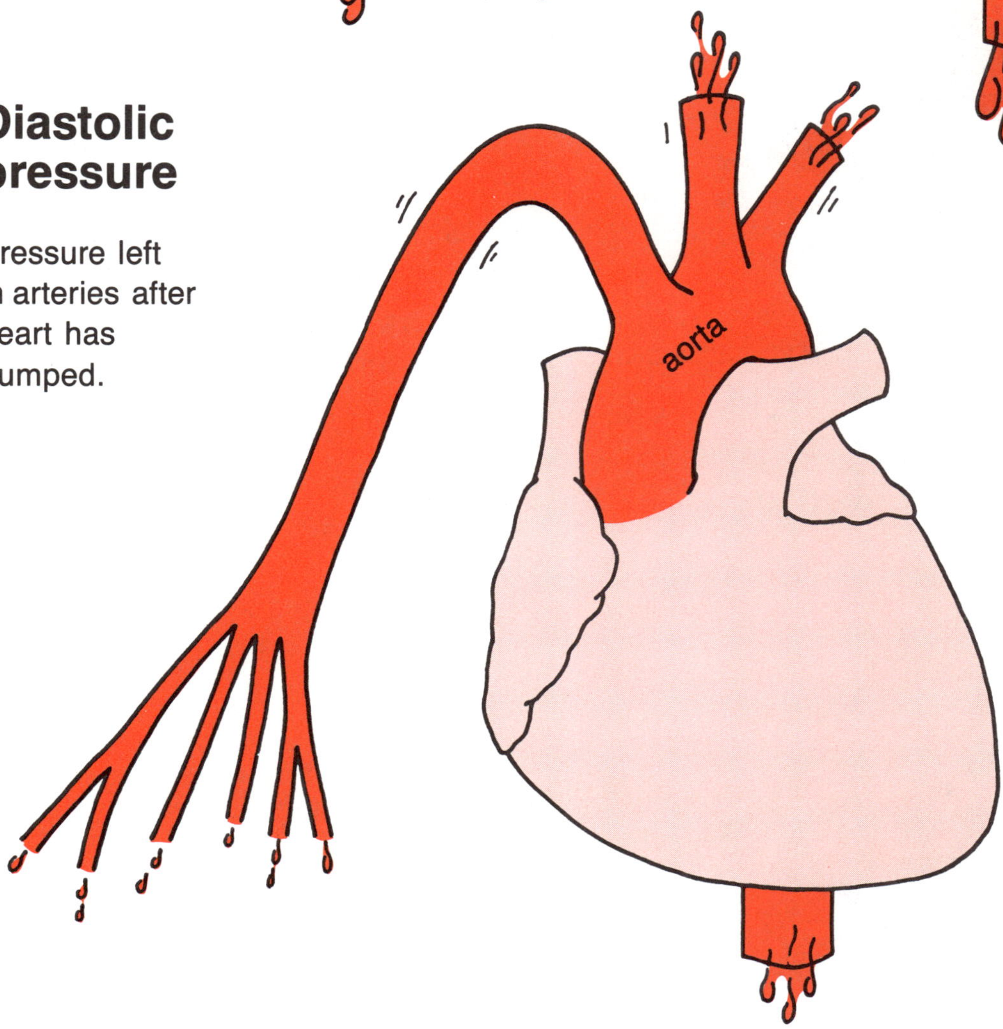

When blood pressure is high

Blood pressure is recorded with a set of 2 numbers such as 140/90. The top number (140) is the systolic pressure, and the bottom number (90) is the diastolic pressure. If 3 or more blood pressure checks in a row show a diastolic (bottom number) pressure higher than 90, it is likely that you have high blood pressure. The degrees of high blood pressure for adults of 18 years and older are:

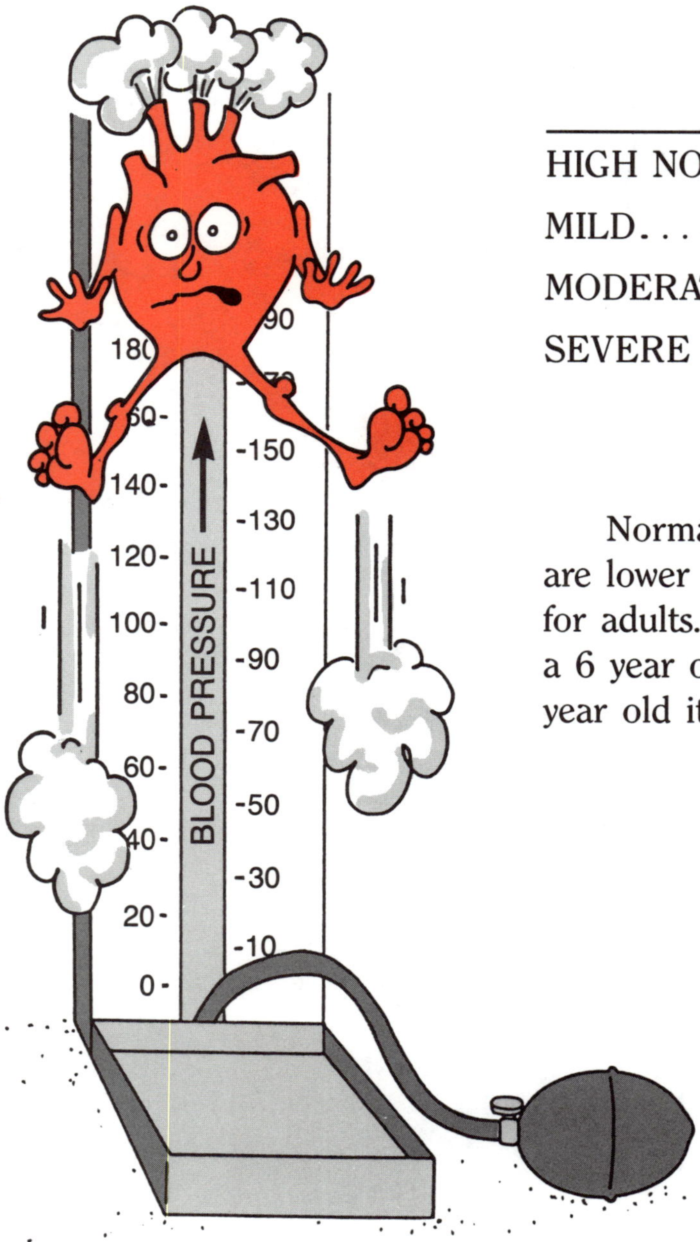

	Diastolic BP (bottom number)
HIGH NORMAL	85 to 89
MILD.	90 to 104
MODERATE	105 to 114
SEVERE	greater than 114

Normal blood pressures for children are lower than normal blood pressures for adults. A normal blood pressure for a 6 year old might be 110/75. For a 14 year old it might be 125/85.

Types of high blood pressure

Ninety percent of people with chronic high blood pressure have what is called **"essential hypertension."** This means there is no known cause. Studies are being done to see:

- if substances put out by the kidneys lead to high blood pressure
- if nerves in the small arteries cause the arteries to tighten
- how diet,* heredity and fluid retention affect blood pressure

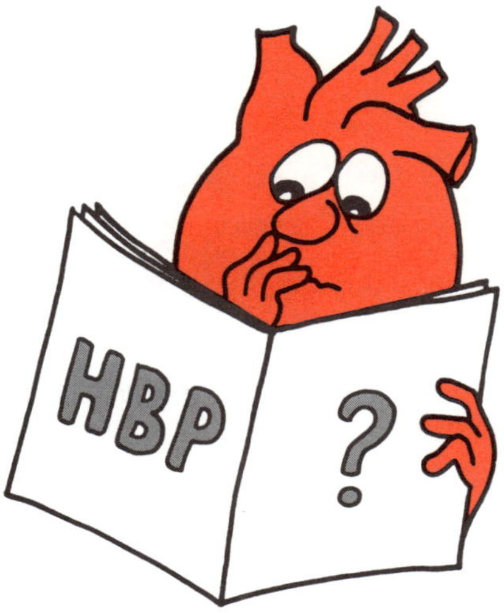

The other 10% of the people with chronic high blood pressure have **"secondary hypertension."** This form of high blood pressure most often comes from problems in the kidneys or renal arteries. It can also be due to glandular tumors.

Some drugs can raise blood pressure at times in some people. (For example: birth control pills, certain arthritis medicines and some "cold" remedies) When such a person stops using these drugs, blood pressure can sometimes go down.

*Research is now being done on calcium and high blood pressure. Studies are looking to see if a diet low in calcium is related to high blood pressure.

People with hypertension

There does seem to be a pattern as to who gets hypertension:

- **Black Americans** are about twice as likely to have it as whites. This could be due to a combination of things like heredity, stress and lifestyle.

- **Children of parents with high blood pressure** are 6 times as likely to get high blood pressure if both parents have it. Children are 4 times as likely to have high blood pressure if one parent has it. High blood pressure often shows up earlier in children of hypertensive parents, sometimes even in the teens.

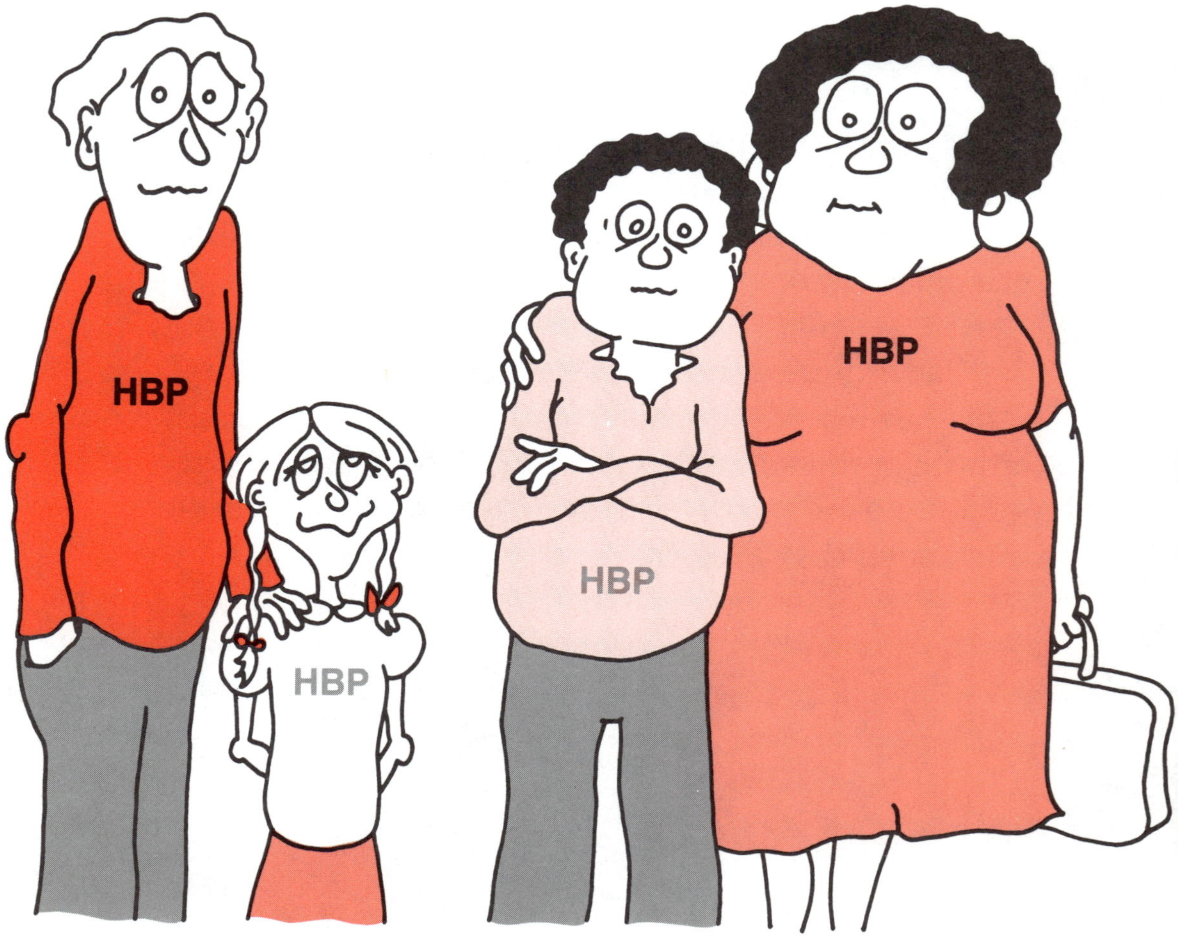

- **Fat people** have hypertension much more often than thin people.

- **Diets** high in salt can make high blood pressure worse.

- People who have poor **health habits** are more likely to have high blood pressure. This would include bad eating habits, drinking too much, being unable to handle stress and not exercising enough.

- **Men are somewhat more likely than women to get high blood pressure** before age 45. But after age 45 women and men have about the same chance of having high blood pressure.

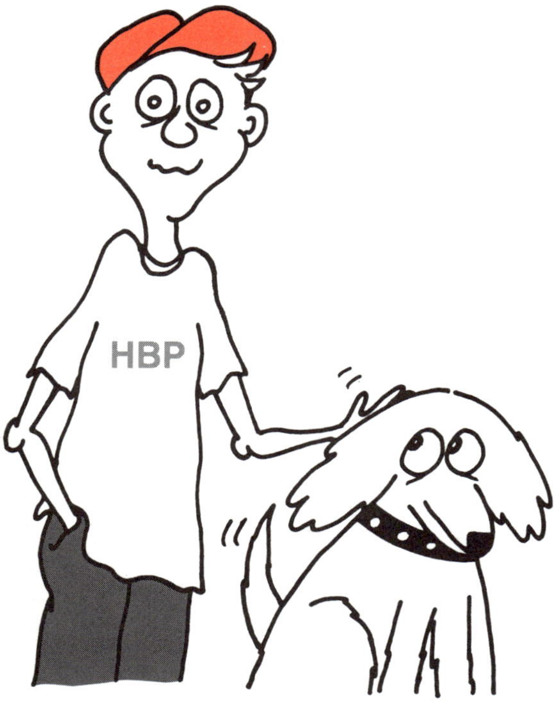

HBP = High Blood Pressure

Treatment

In the next 29 pages you will learn about treatment to control essential hypertension. This will include:

- **what you eat**
- **body weight**
- **medications**
- **relaxation**
- **regular exercise**
- **not smoking**

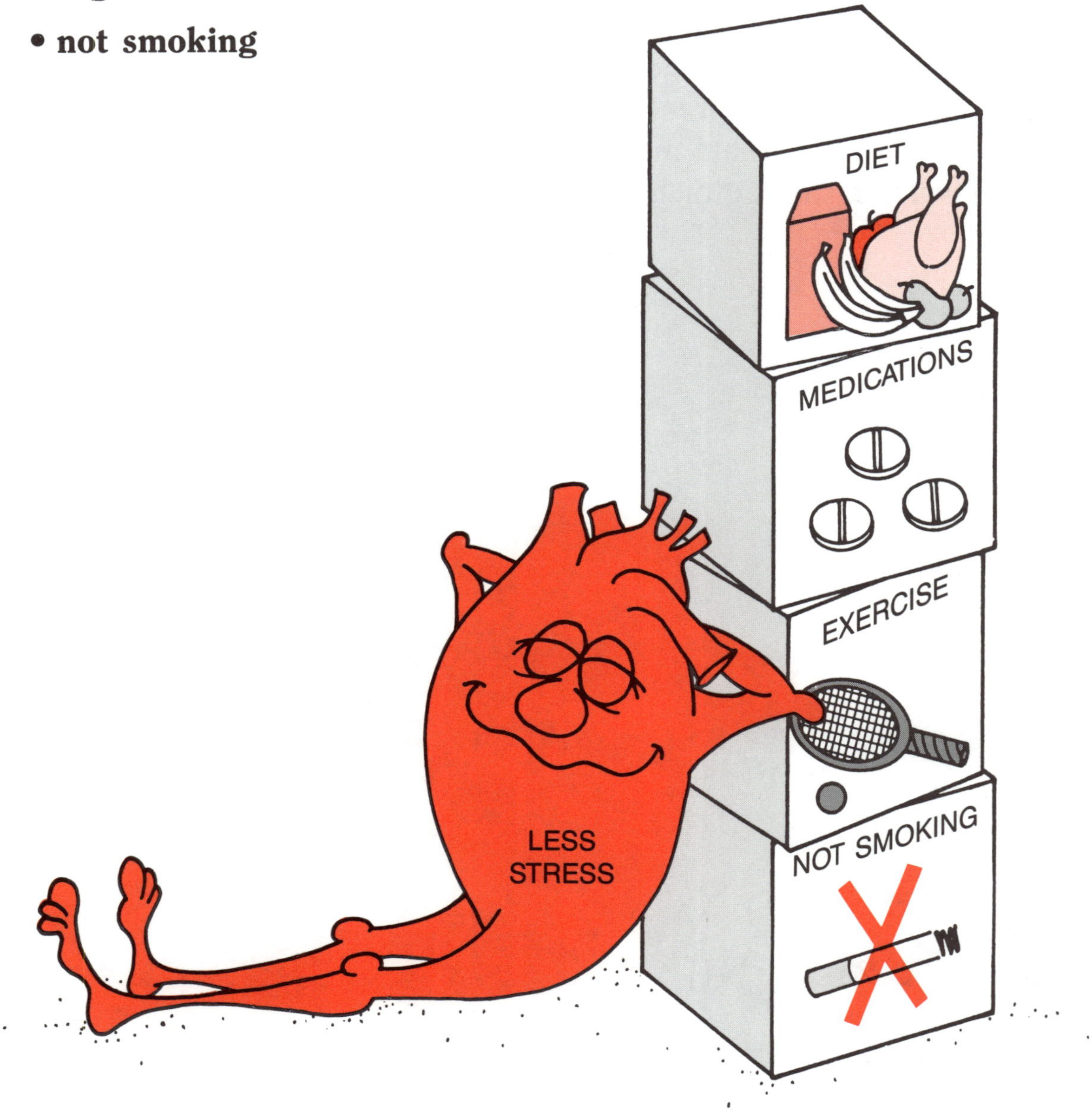

What you eat

Choose foods, drinks and seasonings that are:

- **low in sodium**
- **low in fats and cholesterol**
- **high in potassium**
- **balanced**

The next 18 pages help you buy and prepare foods that promote good health and normal blood pressure. These pages give you only some of the types of foods to eat. Since no 2 bodies are just alike, there is no exact food list for everyone to use. Some people are more sensitive to sodium than others. Some are more prone to a high blood cholesterol than others. On each visit to your doctor, talk about what you are eating. You and your doctor can decide if changes in diet are needed.

If you already eat a balanced, low-sodium, low-fat diet, these food pages will help you keep your good health habits.

If you now eat a lot of salt, "fast" foods or high-fat foods, these food lists may bring out your "moans and groans." At first you may think that you can never eat what you really enjoy. Most likely this won't be true. What will be true, if you are to lower blood pressure, is that fatty, salty foods or drinks will need to be a rare treat. In time, your tastes will change so that you don't crave your old food habits as much.

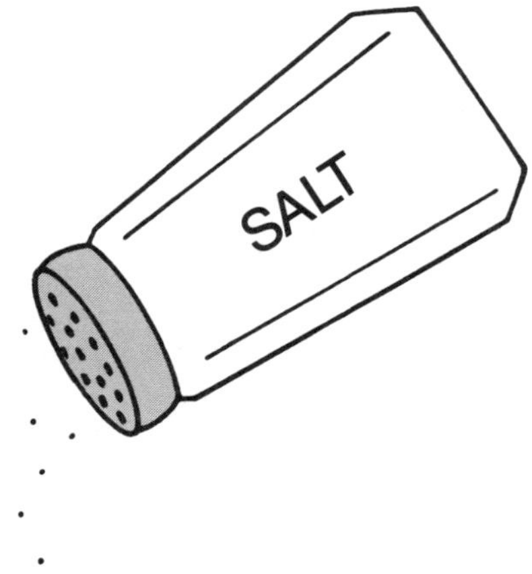

SODIUM is an important mineral. It helps your body balance the level of fluids inside and outside of the cells. To keep up this balance, the body needs little more than 200 mg. of sodium a day. Yet, most of us eat 3,000 to 6,000 mg. of sodium each day. (Our most common source of sodium is table salt.)

For some people extra sodium is no problem. Their kidneys filter and pass excess sodium out of the body into the urine. For others, their kidneys do not filter as well, and some sodium is put back into the blood. This builds up the volume of blood and fluids flowing through the arteries since sodium attracts water. To pump the added fluids, the heart works harder, and blood pressure goes up.

Many people with high blood pressure have a problem with water retention. They are more sensitive to sodium than others.

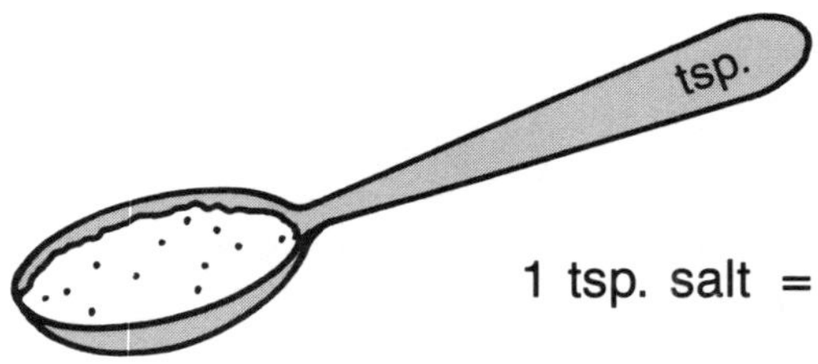

1 tsp. salt = 2,000 mg. sodium

All people with high blood pressure will benefit from a diet of 2,000 mg. of sodium a day or less. (One level teaspoon of salt equals 2,000 mg. of sodium.) We can't prove that too much salt in the diet causes high blood pressure, but we can tell you that in countries where a lot of salt is eaten, blood pressures are the highest.

How to fix low-sodium foods:

- **Rinse foods** before cooking or eating them. This can remove some of the sodium from fresh, frozen or canned foods.

- **Season foods** with fresh dried herbs, vegetables, fruits or no-salt seasonings.

- **Do not cook with salt** or add salt to foods after they are on the table.

- **Make your own** breads, rolls, sauces, salad dressings, vegetable dishes and desserts.

- **Prepare fresh vegetables** when you can. Fresh foods have less sodium than processed foods. For example:*

Instead of:	Use:
1 cup of canned green beans: **320 mg. of sodium**	1 cup of cooked, fresh green beans: **5 mg. of sodium**
1 cup of cooked canned peas: **400 mg. of sodium**	1 cup of fresh, cooked peas: **2 mg. of sodium**
½ cup of Minute® Long Grain and Wild Rice: **570 mg. of sodium**	½ cup of cooked rice: **1 mg. of sodium**

- **Buy water-packed tuna and salmon.** Break up into a bowl of cold water, and let stand for 3 minutes. Rinse, drain and squeeze out water.

- **Bake, broil, boil, steam, roast or poach** meats without salt.

*Sodium contents of foods from USDA Handbook #456.

Low-sodium foods—what to buy

fruits
- fresh, canned or frozen

vegetables
- fresh or frozen
  (no sauce or plastic pouches)

fats, oils*
- canola, olive, corn, cottonseed, peanut, safflower, soybean and sunflower oil
- salad dressing or mayonnaise
  (low-cal and low-sodium)
- margarine (unsalted)

dairy choices*

— liquid or dry milk (1% or skim) — homemade buttermilk (made from powdered milk)	limit to 2-3 cups/day
— cottage cheese, dry curd (low-sodium) — ricotta (made from low-fat or skim milk) — farmer cheese, part-skim mozzarella, neufchatel	limit to ½ cup or 1 oz. of one of these per day

drinks
- fruit juices, fresh or frozen
- canned low-sodium tomato and vegetable juice
- instant breakfast*
  (all flavors but eggnog—limit to 1 cup/day)
- lemonade (frozen concentrate or fresh)
- liquor, wine (not cooking wine)—if allowed
- tea, coffee

meats, poultry, fish
- fish, fresh or frozen (not breaded), canned tuna and salmon
  (unsalted or rinsed—see p. 15)
- chicken or turkey (no skin)
- lean cuts of:
  beef, veal, pork, lamb
- beef tongue

meat substitutes
- dried beans, peas, lentils (not canned)
- nuts or seeds (unsalted, dry roasted)*:
  sunflower seeds, peanuts, almonds, walnuts
- unsalted peanut butter*
- tofu (soybean curd)

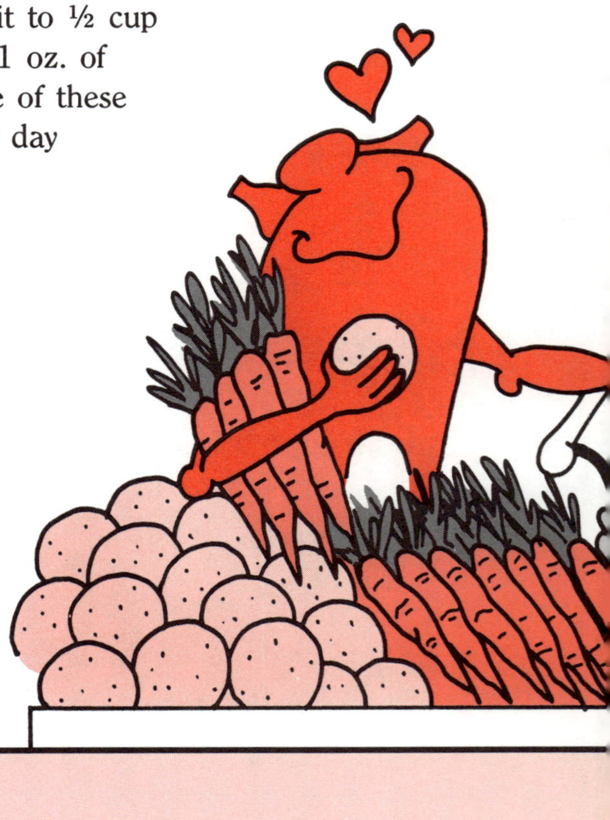

*Contain fairly high amounts of fat and/or calories. Use in small amounts.

breads, cereals, grains, starches

- loaf bread and yeast rolls (limit to 3 slices/day)
- homemade breads (with regular flour, **not** self-rising)
- melba toast
- matzo crackers
- pita bread
- taco shell
- tortilla (corn)
- cooked cereals like: corn grits, farina (regular), oatmeal, oat bran, cream of rice, cream of wheat (do not add salt—avoid **instant** cereals)
- puffed rice or wheat
- shredded wheat
- wheat germ*
- popcorn (no salt or fat added)
- starchy vegetables: corn, potatoes, green peas, etc. (not canned unless salt free)
- rice (enriched white or brown)
- pasta

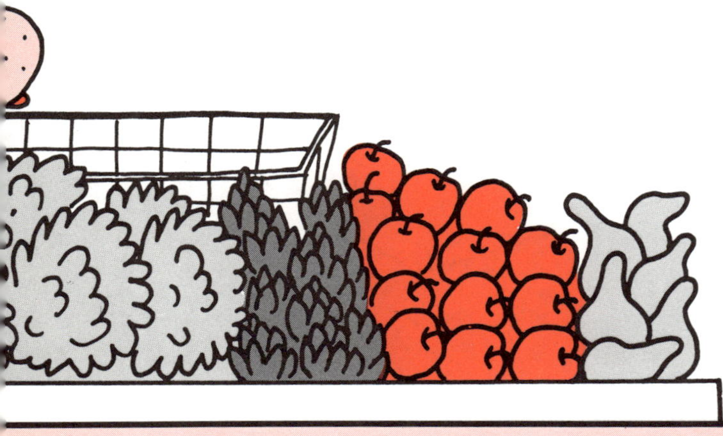

cooking ingredients, seasonings

- corn starch
- corn meal (**not** self-rising)
- dried herbs, salt-free herb seasonings
- flour, regular white or whole wheat (**not** self-rising)
- fresh fruits or vegetables (lemons, limes, onions, celery, etc.)
- fresh garlic or ginger
- Louisiana-type hot sauce (limit to 1 tsp./day)
- low-sodium baking powder
- onion or garlic powder
- tapioca
- tomato paste, unsalted tomatoes, unsalted tomato sauce
- vinegar
- water chestnuts
- yeast

sweets

- carob powder
- cocoa powder
- flavored gelatins (low-calorie)
- fruits (fresh, canned, frozen)
- frozen juice bars, fruit ice, sorbet, sherbet
- sugar, honey, molasses, syrup (cane or maple)
- jelly, jams, preserves, apple butter
- graham & animal crackers, fig bars, ginger snaps

High-sodium foods—AVOID

vegetables
- canned vegetables (unless unsalted)
- sauerkraut

breads, cereals, grains, starches
- self-rising flour and corn meal
- prepared mixes
  (waffle, pancake, muffin, cornbread, etc.)
- instant cooked cereals

dairy products
- buttermilk (store-bought)
- canned milk
  (unless diluted and used as regular milk)
- egg substitute (limit to ½ cup/day)
- eggnog (store-bought)
- salted butter and margarine

soups
- bouillon (all kinds)
- canned broth
- dry soup mixes
- canned soups

meats and meat substitutes
- canned meats
- canned fish
  (sardines, unrinsed tuna and salmon)
- cured meats
  (dried beef, bacon, corned beef, etc.)
- all types sausage
  (beef, pork, chicken, turkey, Polish sausage, hot dogs, knockwurst, etc.)
- sandwich meats
  (bologna, salami, olive loaf, etc.)
- peanut butter
- salted nuts

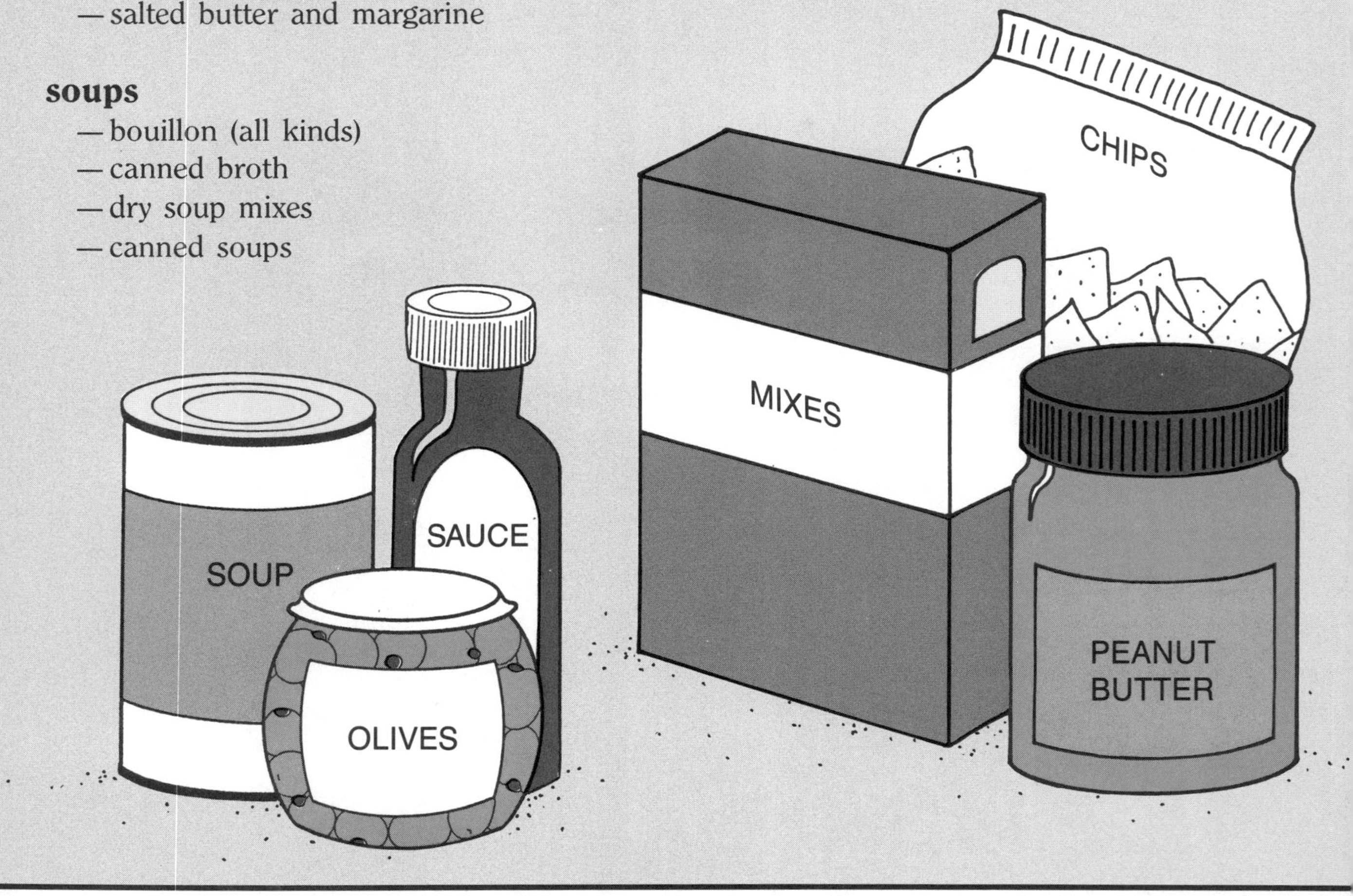

sweets

- prepared mixes (pie, pudding, cake)
- store-bought pies, cakes, muffins

cooking ingredients, seasonings, condiments, snacks

- fermented miso
- preseasoned mixes for tacos, spaghetti, chili, etc.
- coating mixes
- preseasoned convenience foods
- tomato sauce (unless unsalted)
- catsup
- chili sauce
- barbeque sauce
- mustard
- salad dressing

(catsup, chili sauce, barbeque sauce, mustard, salad dressing: use low-sodium type or limit to 2 Tbsp./day)

- baking soda, baking powder (use low-sodium type)
- olives
- pickles (dill, sour, sweet gherkins)
- pretzels, chips, skins, etc.
- soy sauce, teriyaki sauce
- cooking wine
- light salt, seasoning salt, sea salt, meat tenderizer, garlic salt, monosodium glutamate (MSG), celery salt, onion salt, lemon pepper

drinks

- athletic drinks (Thirst Quencher®, Gatorade®)
- canned tomato or vegetable juice (unless unsalted)

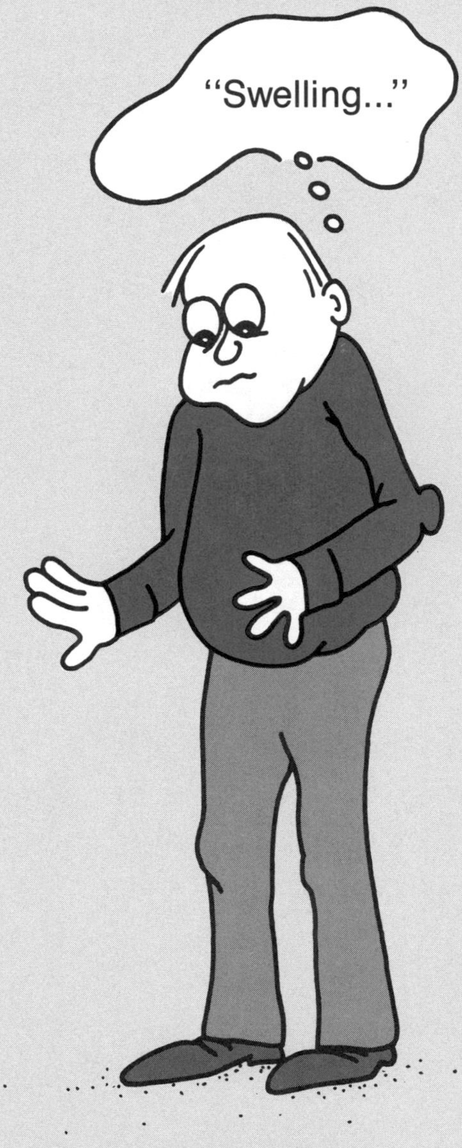

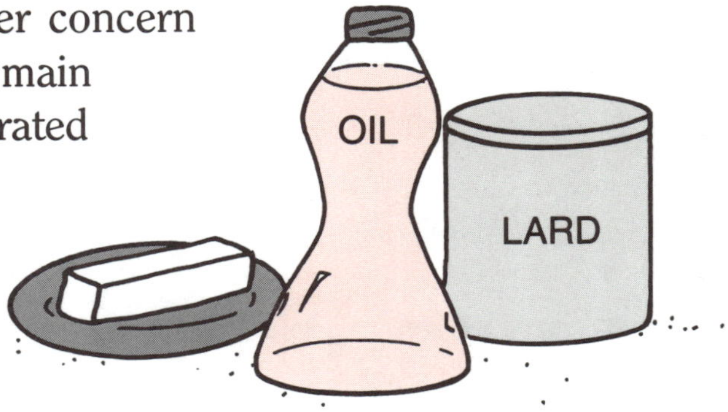

FATS and **CHOLESTEROL** are another concern for people with hypertension. There are 3 main kinds of fat in foods: saturated, polyunsaturated and monounsaturated fats. The fat most harmful to your body is saturated fat. Saturated fat and cholesterol in foods can raise blood cholesterol levels.

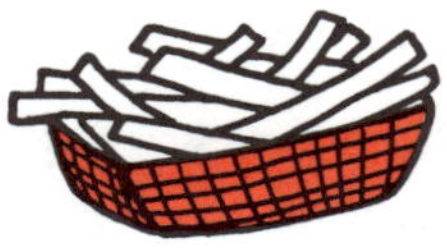

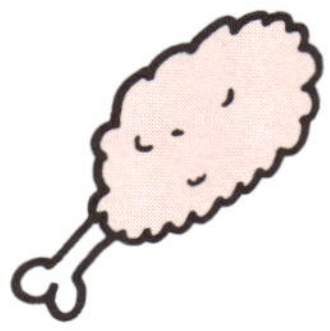

Having high blood cholesterol levels puts you at risk for heart disease. When there is too much cholesterol in the blood, a fatty plaque builds up on the artery walls, and the arteries become narrow. If blood can't pass through the clogged artery to the heart, a heart attack or stroke will occur.

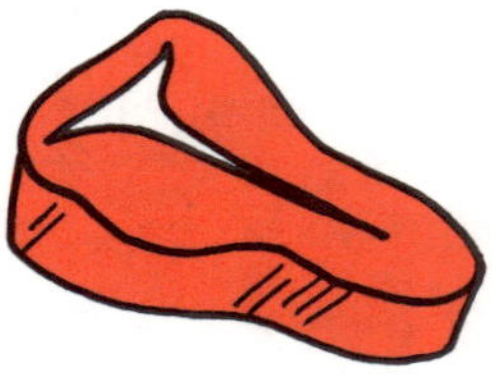

You can help prevent this buildup in the blood vessels by eating low-fat, low-cholesterol foods. Eating these types of foods is even more important when it is known that heart disease runs in your family. The earlier you change your diet, the more likely you are to avoid a heart attack or stroke.

The American Heart Association suggests that you get no more than 30% of your daily calories from fats. Less than 10% should come from saturated fat, up to 10% from polyunsaturated fat and the rest from monounsaturated fat. To stay within this limit, avoid foods listed as high-fat, high-cholesterol (p. 24), and use the tips on page 21 for preparing foods.

How to fix low-fat, low-cholesterol foods:

- **Bake, broil, boil, steam, roast or poach** foods. Serve without fatty sauces. Don't fry. Use very little oil when stir frying. A vegetable oil spray, used lightly, will keep foods from sticking to the pan.

- **Cook more fish and poultry** (light meat). Eat lean, red meats only 3-4 times a week. Trim off all excess fat before cooking. Remove skin from chicken and turkey.

- **Drain all meats** on a paper towel after cooking. The towel will soak up extra grease or fat.

- **Season foods with herbs, fruits and vegetables.** Do not cook with saturated fat (butter, lard, ham hocks, fatback, sausages).

- **Cook with small amounts of vegetable oils** (polyunsaturated or monounsaturated). Use 1 Tbsp. or less per dish. Make salad dressings with small amounts of polyunsaturated or monounsaturated oil.

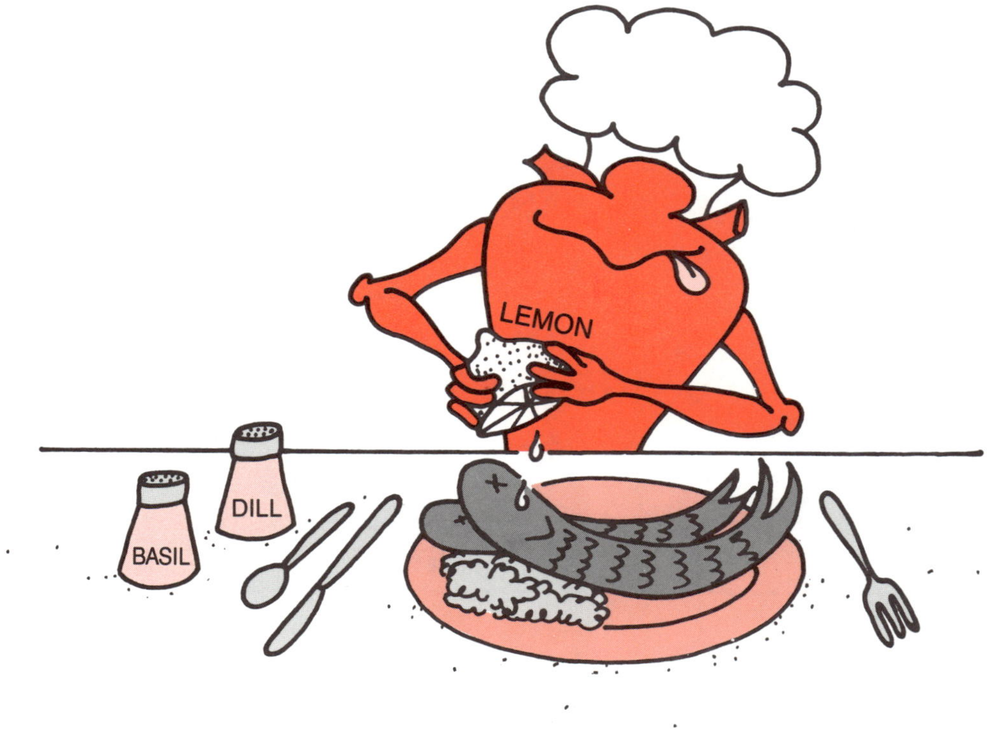

Low-fat, low-cholesterol foods—what to buy

fruits, vegetables

— any fresh, frozen (no sauces or pouches) or canned (unsalted)

breads, cereals, grains, starches

— bagels
— English muffins*
— enriched plain flour, plain corn meal
— homemade breads (with vegetable oil), store-bought breads (limit to 3 slices/day)
— air popcorn (or popcorn made with small amounts of vegetable oil)
— pita bread
— starchy vegetables (corn, potatoes, green peas, etc.)
— tortillas
— whole grain or white enriched bread, cereal, rice, pasta (oat bran, oatmeal, wheat or bran breads or cereal, brown rice, plain macaroni, noodles)

milk choices

(1% milk fat or less—limit to 2-3 cups/day)

— buttermilk* (store-bought)
— evaporated skim milk (limit to ½ cup/day)
— nonfat or low-fat yogurt
— nonfat dry milk
— skim or liquid nonfat milk

cheeses

(limit to 1 oz./day unless low-sodium and low-fat)

— farmer
— part-skim mozzarella
— parmesan*
— ricotta or uncreamed cottage (1% milk fat—limit to ½ cup/day)

convenience foods

— canned or dried soups made with clear broth (low-sodium types)

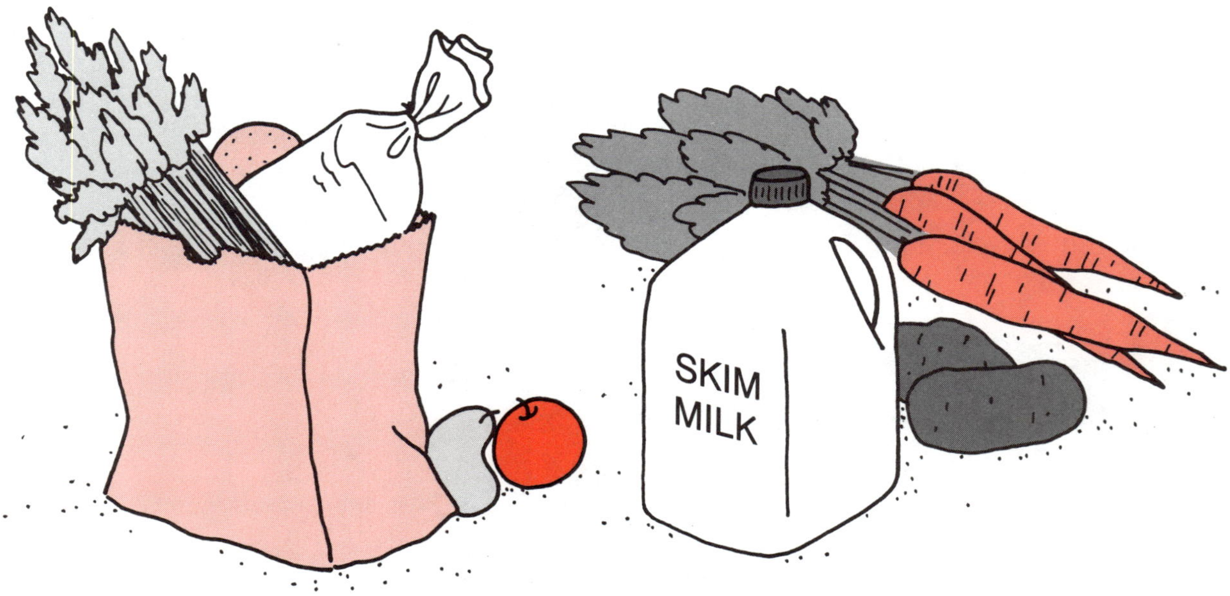

*Avoid if you need to eat less sodium.

†Recent research suggests that cold water fish such as salmon, mackeral and tuna contain Omega 3 fatty acids which may help reduce the risk of heart disease. The American Heart Associ-

meats, poultry, fish
- all fish (includes tuna or salmon packed in water and rinsed)†
- fresh chicken or turkey (light meat without skin)
- lean meats (closely trimmed of fat)
  beef: (eye round steak and roast; rump and top round roast; tip steak and roast; lean cubed, top loin, flank and T-bone steaks; tenderloin steak and roast; sirloin; chuck; ground—90% lean)
  veal: (cutlet, leg, rump, shank, shoulder, steak)
  pork: (fresh, uncured cuts)
  lamb: (shank, shoulder)
- scallops, clams, oysters

meat substitutes
- dried beans, peas, lentils
- egg whites (unlimited)
- egg yolks (limit to 2-3/week, including those used in cooking)
- tofu (soybean curd)

fats, oils
(use small amounts; not a low-fat food, but low in saturated fat and low or without cholesterol)
- canola, olive, corn, cottonseed, peanut, safflower, sunflower and soybean oil
- salad dressing or mayonnaise with polyunsaturated or monounsaturated oil
- soft margarines that list liquid polyunsaturated oil first

seasonings, condiments
- dried herbs
- wine
- fresh fruits or vegetables
- fresh garlic or ginger
- horseradish
- ketchup
- mayonnaise
- mustard

(ketchup, mayonnaise, mustard: low-sodium or limit to 2 Tbsp./day)

- onion or garlic powder
- vinegar

sweets
(depending on need for weight control)
- angel food cake
- carob powder
- cocoa powder
- flavored gelatins
- fresh fruits
- frozen juice bars, fruit ice, sorbet, sherbet
- low-fat frozen milk desserts (with less than 3 gm. fat/serving)
- graham & animal crackers, fig bars, ginger snaps
- sugar, honey, jams, jellies

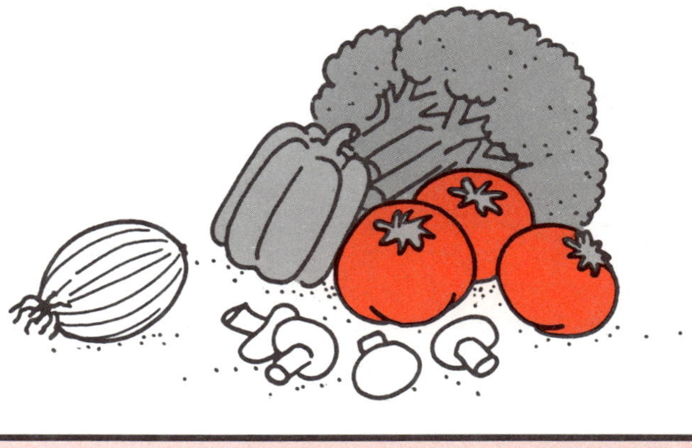

ation (AHA) suggests limiting shrimp, lobster and sardines* to one 3 oz. serving per week. The AHA does not recommend the use of fish oil supplements.

High-fat and/or high-cholesterol foods— AVOID

- saturated fats
  (butter, lard, meat fats)
- hydrogenated or partially hydrogenated fats*
  (shortening, even if it says "no cholesterol")
- coconut, palm or palm kernel oils
- whole milk dairy products
- cream, sour cream, whipping cream
- creamed cheese or cheddar, Swiss, Roquefort, blue, camembert, brie, any whole milk cheese
- croissants, cheese breads, egg breads, biscuits, high-fat crackers (those that feel oily)
- store-bought cakes, pies, doughnuts, cookies
- egg yolks (see p. 23)
- caviar, roe, fish eggs
- fried foods
- dark meat of poultry
- domestic duck, goose
- hot dogs, knockwurst, Polish sausage, etc.
- liver, brains, sweetbreads, kidney, heart, chitterlings
- red meats (beef, lamb, pork, veal) with a lot of fatty streaks in them
- oil-packed canned tuna, salmon and sardines

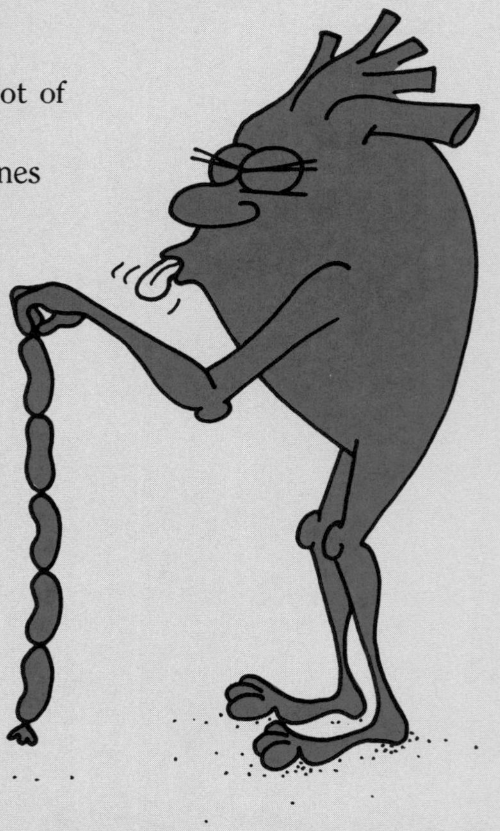

*When a fat is "hydrogenated," it stays more solid at room temperature. Companies that make margarine and cooking oils may add hydrogen to the fat content to make the product more like a saturated fat.

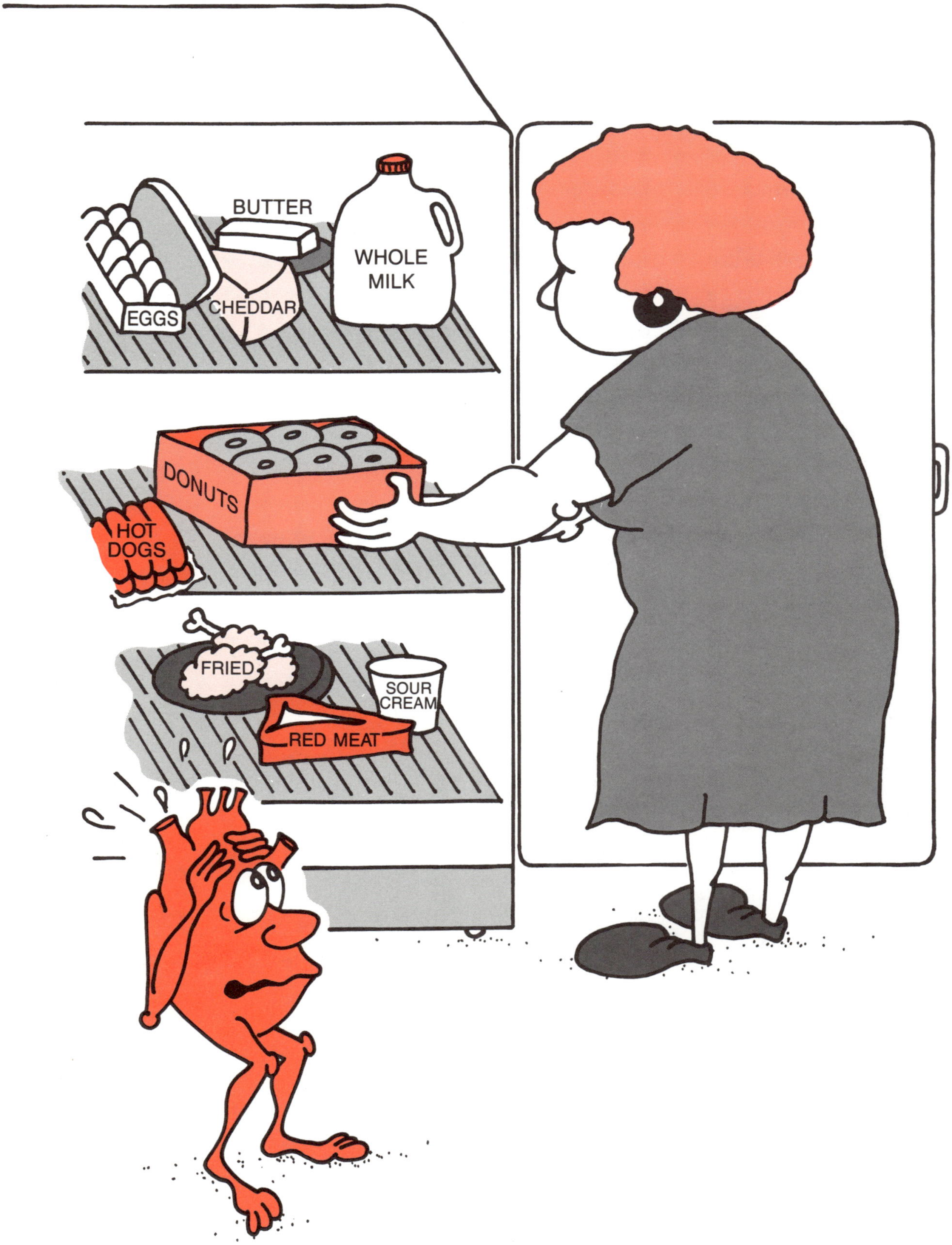
BUTTER
WHOLE MILK
EGGS
CHEDDAR
DONUTS
HOT DOGS
FRIED
SOUR CREAM
RED MEAT

Like sodium, **POTASSIUM** is an important mineral. It helps regulate your heart rhythm. Without enough potassium, you may have:

- irregular heartbeats
- muscle weakness and cramps
- dizzy spells
- fatigue

If you are taking a diuretic (water pill) for fluid retention, you may need to eat more potassium and/or take a potassium supplement. You need to prevent the loss of too much potassium when fluids pass out of the body. Ask your doctor about potassium if he or she prescribes a diuretic. **Do not** take a potassium supplement unless your doctor prescribes it.

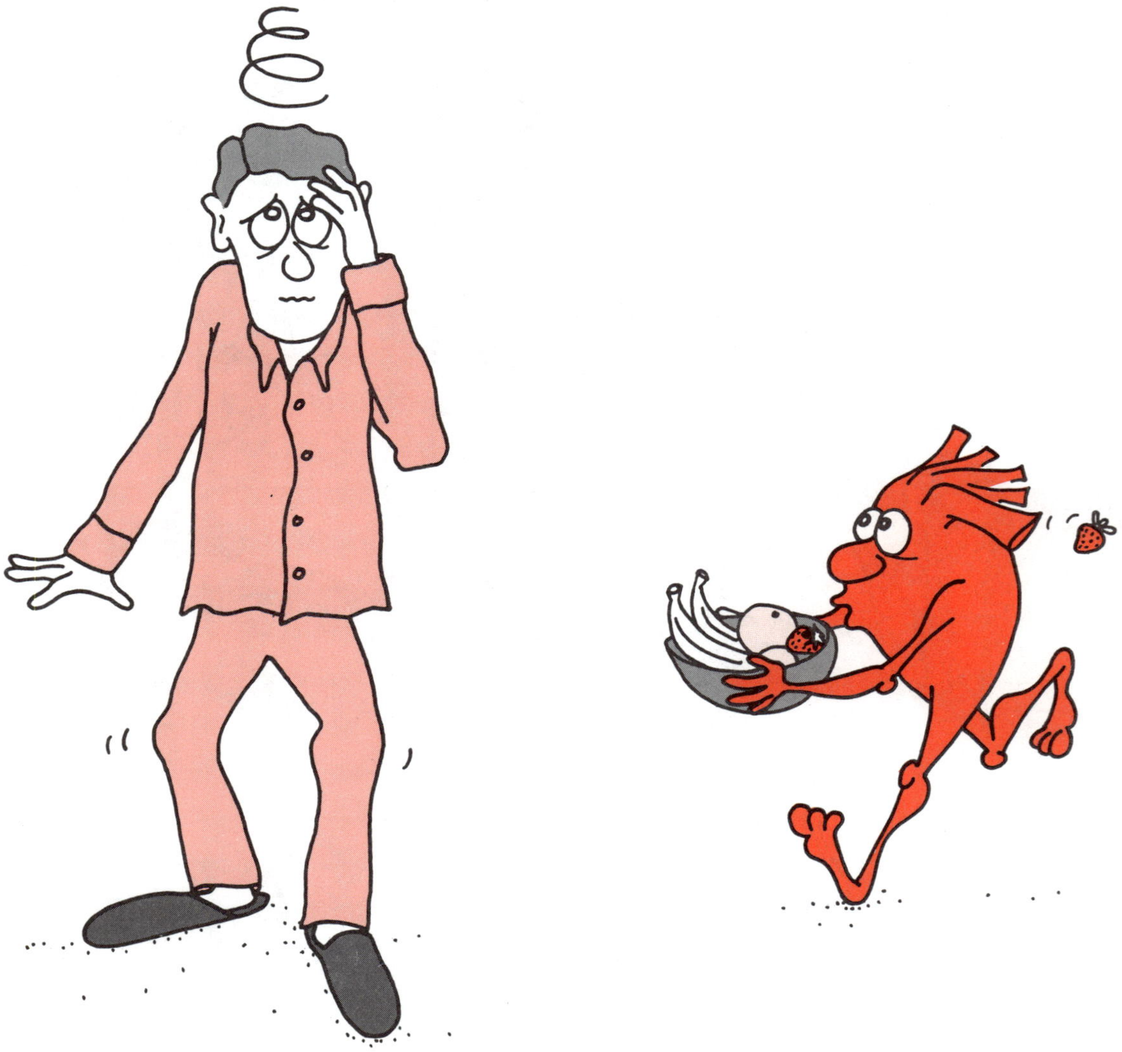

High-potassium foods—what to buy

fruits
- apricots
- avocados
- bananas
- cantaloupe
- dates
- fruit cocktail
- grapefruit
- honeydew melon
- oranges
- peaches
- prunes
- raisins
- strawberries
- watermelon

vegetables
- artichokes
- broccoli
- Brussels sprouts
- carrots
- greens
- squash
- sweet potatoes
- tomatoes
- white potatoes

milk choices
- milk, all kinds (best to use skim)

meats & meat substitutes
- beef
- fresh pork
- chicken
- turkey
- fish
- cooked dried beans
- peanuts

juices
- grapefruit
- orange
- pineapple
- prune
- unsalted tomato or vegetable

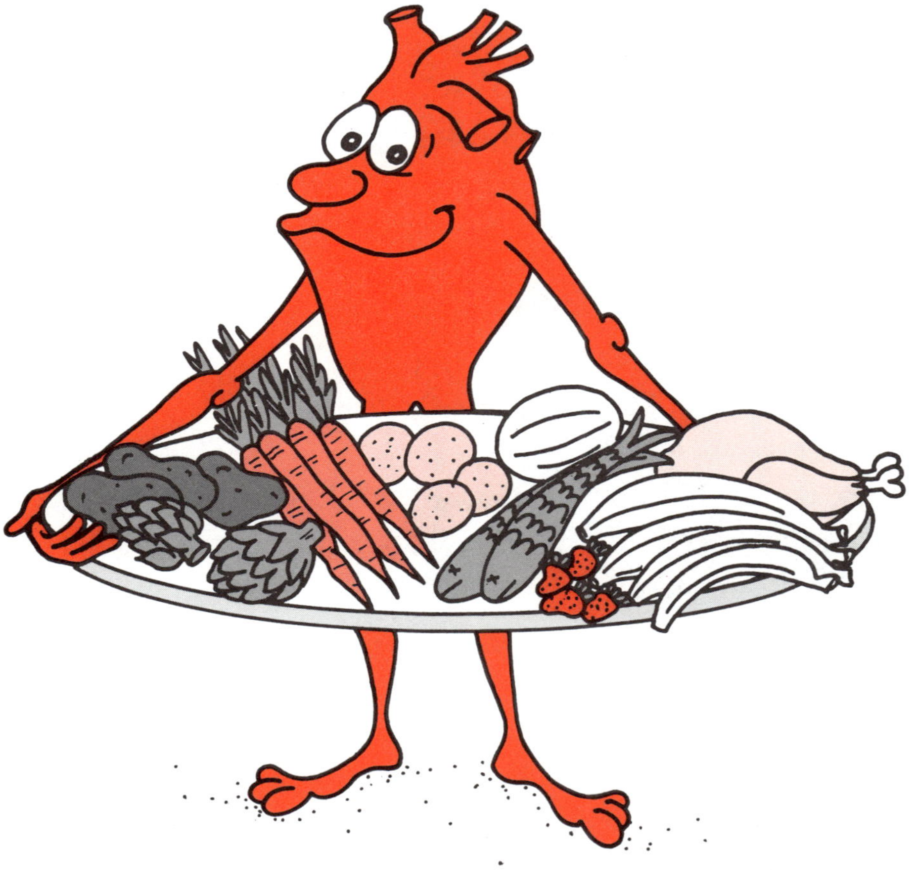

Balanced meals

To stay healthy, you need to eat foods from each of the 6 basic food groups each day.

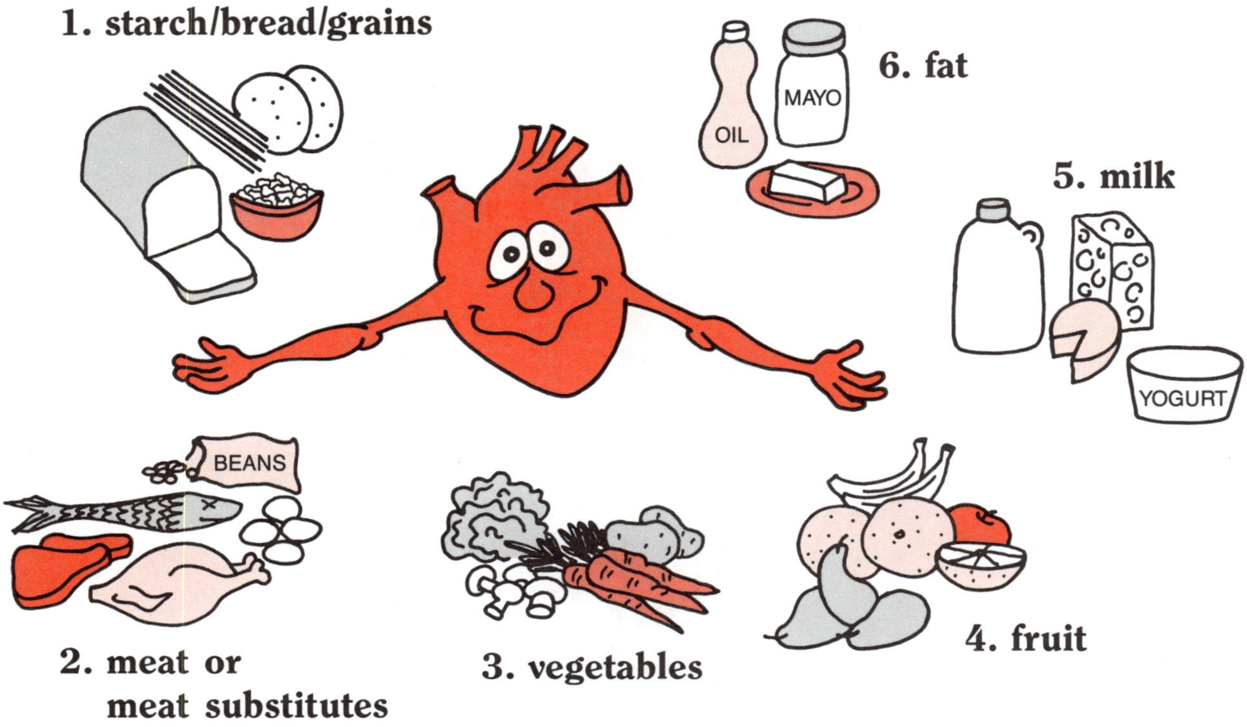

No one food group can give your body all that it needs. It is a balance of many foods that makes you feel good and stay healthy.

If you stick to serving sizes, you can eat many kinds of foods and control weight. Most food labels will tell you how many servings are in a can or package. Here are some amounts that equal one serving:

½ cup peas	1-6″ banana
1 cup melon cubes	1 medium sized potato
4 to 6 crackers	3 to 4 oz. beef
1 cup skim milk	1 tsp. cooking oil
1 medium fish fillet	1 oz. farmer cheese

Food labels

One way to buy foods with less fat, cholesterol, sodium or sugar is to **read all food labels.**

Some products may say, "No cholesterol," "made with 100% vegetable oil" or "99% fat free" on the front label. But when you read the fine print on the back you may see that the product is high in saturated fat. You need to compare grams of fat on the label. For example, one cheese product may have 9 gms. of fat per serving while another may have 3 gms. of fat. But if you read a vegetable oil label, it may have 14 gms. of fat per serving. So each food can only to be compared with another food of the same kind.

The sugar content is often not listed in grams. If sugar is the 1st or 2nd item listed on a label, the product is most likely over 50% sugar. (Dextrose, fructose, sucrose, honey, molasses, brown or raw sugar and sorbitol all count as sugar.)

Buy foods that list 140 mg. of sodium or less on the label. This list will help you to read sodium labels:*

• **sodium free**	5 mg. or less sodium/serving
• **very low sodium**	35 mg. or less/serving
• **low sodium**	140 mg. or less/serving
• **reduced sodium**	1 serving has no more than 75% of the sodium in the regular product (this can still be high in sodium)
• **no salt added, unsalted, without added salt**	no salt added during processing (only used for foods that usually have salt added)

*Definitions provided by the Food and Drug Administration.

Mystery foods

Eating out is a problem when you want to eat less fat, sodium or sugar. You can't always tell what is in a dish. And even if you ask that foods be fixed a certain way, you can't be sure it was done as you asked. To get around this problem, do these:

- Order any salad dressing on the side; put only 1 Tbsp. of it on your salad.

- Order fish or poultry (light meat); ask that it be broiled, baked, roasted or poached (without sauces or butter). Eat red meats at home where you can control the fat.

- Order baked potatoes plain.

- Do not eat real butter. Eat only one pat of margarine.

- Order vegetables without sauces or breading.

- Kill some of your appetite before you go out. Eat a healthy snack such as a large piece of fruit, glass of skim milk, crackers and low-fat cheese or a handful of carrot sticks.

Alcohol (for those who can have it)

Drink no more than 2 servings of alcohol in any one day. This means no more than 2 oz. of 80 proof whiskey or 7 oz. of wine or 24 oz. of beer.* Alcohol does not cause heart attacks, as some people think, but a lot of alcohol can cause skipped heartbeats. Too much alcohol can also weaken the heart muscle and raise blood pressure.

*If beer is 4% alcohol or less

Snacks

Everyone snacks at some time. The best snacks for weight control and blood pressure control would be foods or drinks such as these:

- fresh fruit
- raw vegetables
- dips made with low-fat or nonfat yogurt
- popcorn without oil or salt (try using a vegetable oil spray and adding powdered, fat-free butter granules)
- angel food cake
- fruit sorbets, fruit bars, sherbet, frozen fruit yogurt (low-fat)
- fig bars (4 or 5)
- ginger snaps (4 or 5)
- graham crackers (2 or 3)
- unsalted pretzels
- sodas made with diet drinks and ice milk or sherbet

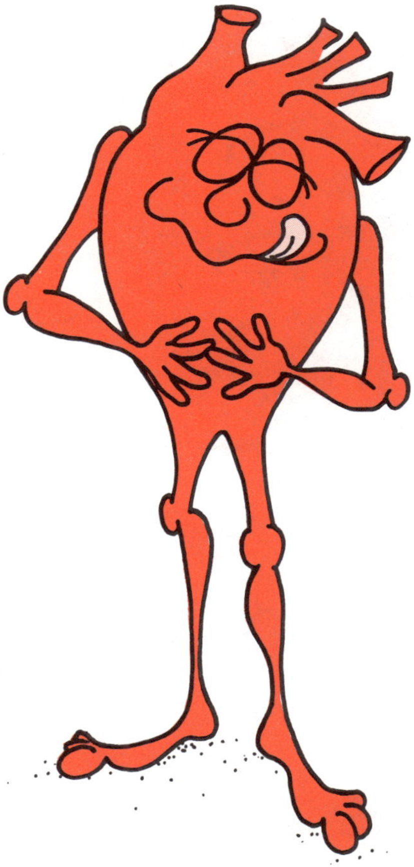

Body weight

If you weigh 10 to 20% more than you should, your doctor will most likely tell you to lose weight. Weight loss lightens the work of the heart and helps high blood pressure to come down.

Choose a diet that lets you lose weight slowly. Your doctor or a registered dietitian can suggest one. Do not choose diets that claim a "quick fix" of fast weight loss in a short time. In the long run, these diets can make weight loss harder. Very low-calorie diets can even be dangerous for people taking a drug to lower blood pressure.

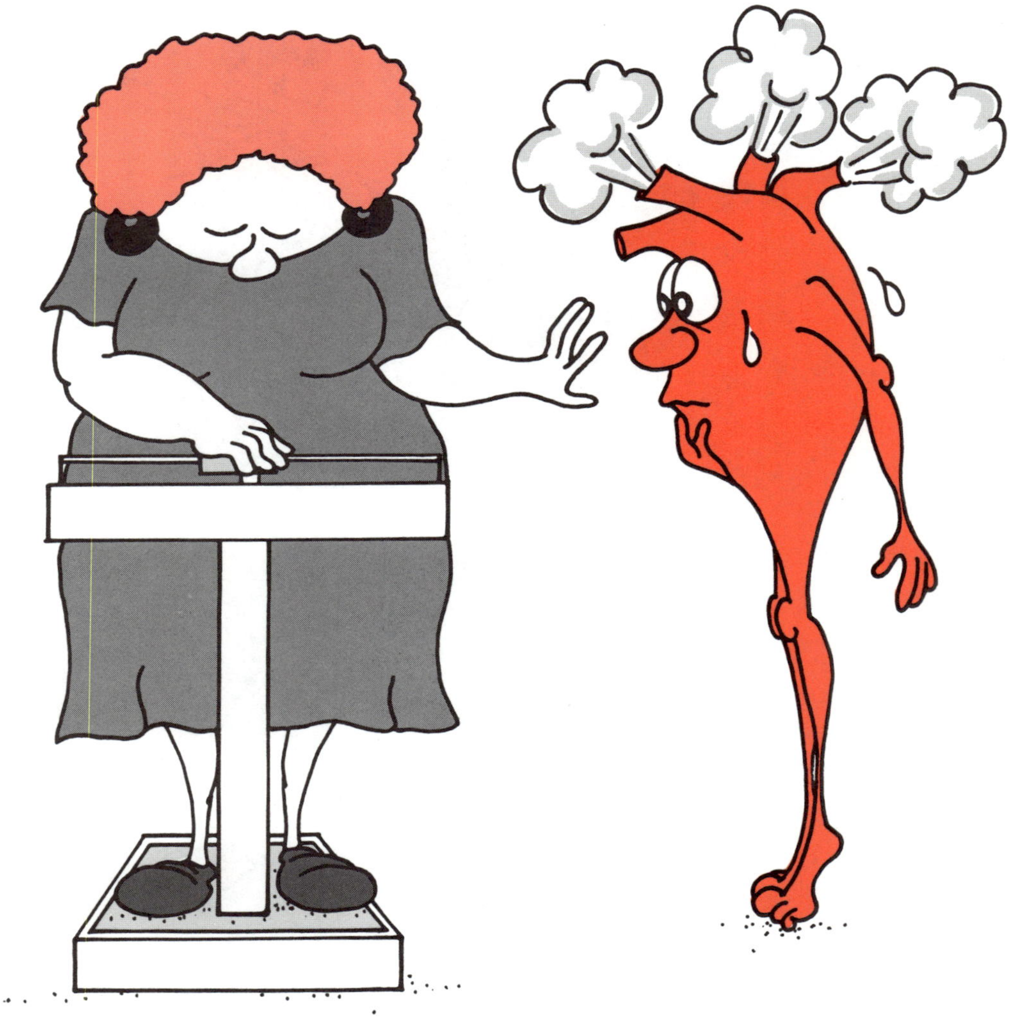

Good diets help you lose weight slowly without losing your health. On a good diet you learn what to eat and in what amounts. Your body thinks "all is well," and weight comes off and stays off. Regular exercise at the same time makes a good diet work even better. Here are some choices to help you get started.

- Choose a diet that allows a good variety of foods from all the basic food groups (p. 28).

- Find a good cookbook or two that contain healthy, tasty recipes for some foods that you like (inside back cover).

- Watch the fats and oils. Salads are great, but salad dressings are very high in fat (and calories).

- Drinks sweetened with sugar are high in calories. Stick with those made with artificial sweetener.

- Choose fruits canned in juice or water rather than syrup. Use sugar-free gelatin. Use only small amounts of jelly, jam, preserves, honey, etc. (Try the "lighter" versions.)

- Limit alcohol, and avoid sweet mixed drinks. (Check with your doctor before drinking alcohol if you are on a medication for your blood pressure.)

There is no magic formula for losing weight. But if you change your eating habits to moderate servings of low-fat, low-sugar foods, you can lose weight and keep it off for life.

Medications

When blood pressure is around 160/95 or above, most doctors will prescribe a drug to help you lower it. Many people stay on a blood pressure medication for life. Others only take pills for awhile. It depends on how well the other parts of your treatment work. So if a drug is prescribed, it may be one or more of these:

- **diuretic** (water pill that helps the body get rid of excess salt and fluid)
- **beta-blocker** (slows down the heart rate; helps keep the heart from beating too vigorously)
- **calcium channel blocker** (keeps artery muscles from squeezing down)
- **vasodilator** (relaxes artery muscles and opens blood vessels)
- **central agent** (acts on the brain to slow down the release of substances that cause arteries to tighten)
- **peripheral neural inhibitor** (acts on the nerves outside the brain to help keep arteries open)
- **alpha blocker** (like the above, it acts on the nerves outside the brain to keep the arteries open)
- **converting enzyme inhibitor** (blocks the making of "angiotensin"; this is a body chemical that promotes artery constriction)

Ask your doctor or druggist how your medication works to help you lower blood pressure. Write the drug name here and what it does for you. ____________________

____

____

℞

Always take your medication just as your doctor prescribes. If there are side effects from the drug, be sure to let your doctor know right away. He or she may need to change the dose or change to another drug. Be patient. Sometimes you may have to try 2 or 3 drugs before finding the right one for you—one that lowers your blood pressure without unpleasant side effects.

Also, as changes occur in your life, (moves, marriage, divorce, children, job changes, weight gain, etc.), the added stress may cause a need for an increase in your medicine for a time. When this happens, your doctor will adjust your medicine to keep your blood pressure within the desired range.

There are some changes (losing weight, reducing sodium in your diet, lowering stress) that may mean your doctor could reduce your medication or even stop it. But **never reduce the dose or stop taking your medicine unless your doctor tells you to.**

And never, EVER take anyone else's medicine or let anyone take yours!

Over-the-counter-drugs

People with high blood pressure should **use over-the-counter drugs only as directed by a doctor.** Some non-prescription drugs contain sodium or vasoconstrictors. Vasoconstrictors can raise blood pressure by causing blood vessels to become more narrow.

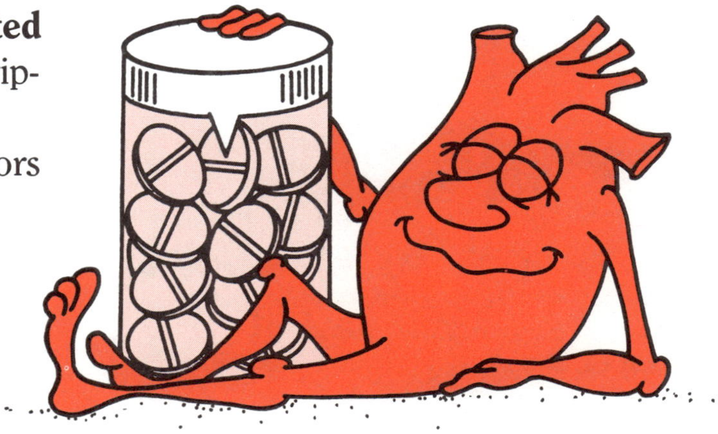

Relaxation

Research has shown that relaxation can help lower blood pressure a little in some people. But relaxation only works for blood pressure when it is done every day along with your other treatment. Here are 2 relaxation methods that have helped a lot of people manage stress.

One way to relax (plan for 20 minutes)

1. **Sit or lie quietly** in a comfortable position away from interruptions (TV, radio, pets, children, phone, etc.)

2. **Close your eyes.**

3. Begin to **relax each muscle** of your body, working up from the feet to the face. Don't rush. When you feel no tightness, stay quiet and still.

4. **Breathe easily** through your nose. Become aware of your breathing. Each time you exhale, repeat the word "one."*

5. When you feel that it is time to come out of this relaxed state, open your eyes slowly. Sit quietly for a minute before getting up.

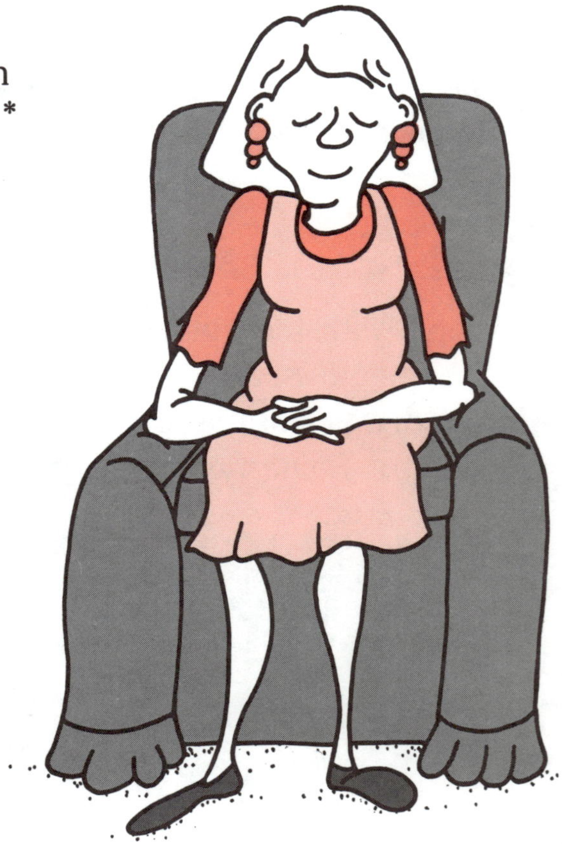

*This method comes from *The Relaxation Response,* by Herbert Benson, M.D., with Miriam Z. Klipper, © 1975; paperback or hardback; Avon Books, publisher; available in major bookstores.

Another way to relax (plan for 20 minutes)

1. Sit or lie quietly in a **comfortable place** where you can't be disturbed. In many homes, this is a hard place to find, but do your best.

2. Close your eyes. Take a few **slow, deep breaths.** As you breathe out, let your body go loose. Release the tightness. Breathe slowly and easily.

3. Think of a time or place that was **a lot of fun** for you. Think about everything that went on that made it fun. Remember the sounds, smells, feelings or people that may have been there.

4. Continue to relax and think of this fun time. If you really **lose yourself in this memory,** your body will begin to relax.

5. As your private time comes to an end, **open your eyes slowly.** Lie or sit quietly for a few minutes before getting up. **Plan another quiet time for tomorrow.**

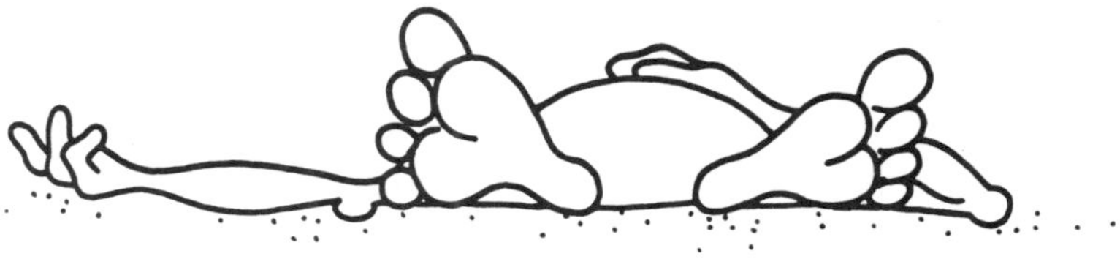

About relaxation

When you first practice relaxation, both body and mind release stress. The release may bring tears, joy or anger. If an emotion wells up, just "go with the flow." It's your private time, and what happens in your time is OK.

A quiet time of 20 minutes is suggested, but don't let tension about time keep you from being able to relax. The more you practice relaxation the longer you will want to be in your quiet place.

Regular exercise

The overall result of regular, non-competitive exercise is that high blood pressure often improves. This is due to:

- a loss of body fat
- a gain in muscle tone and strength (including that of the heart)
- toning of the blood vessels, making them less stiff
- improved blood flow
- stress release and better self-image
- sweat and the loss of excess salt from the body
- less blood fat or buildup (atherosclerosis) in the arteries

Since you have high blood pressure, your doctor should prescribe the amount and type of exercise that is safe for you. Most often blood pressure will have to be controlled before you add exercise to your treatment. Your doctor may also suggest that you join a medically supervised exercise program for the best results.

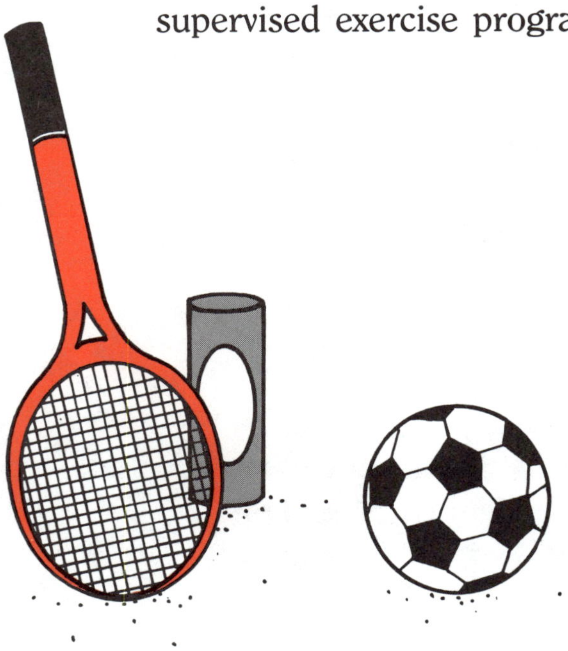

Some kinds of exercise are good for you, and some are bad. Choose the ones that are aerobic and isotonic. Aerobic exercise increases your heart rate and brings oxygen into the body. Walking, jogging, running, dancing and swimming are good aerobic exercises. Calisthenics or yoga would both be isotonic. Do not do isometric exercise without your doctor's OK. Isometric exercises involve strain. Weight lifting and push-ups are isometric. They raise blood pressure while the moves are being done and may not be good for you.

Warming up before exercise and stretching and cooling down afterwards will also be part of any good exercise.

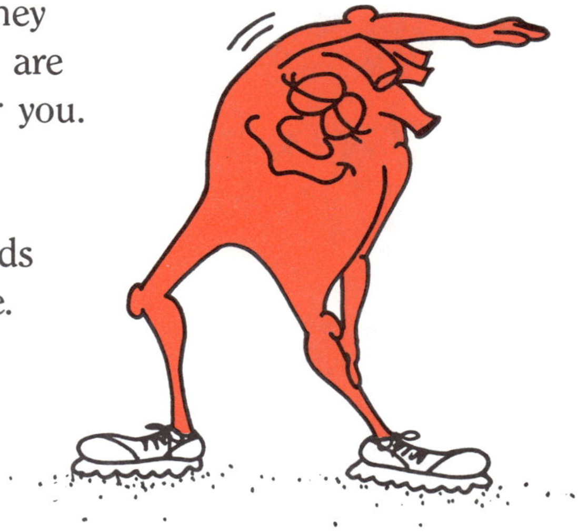

Warm Up

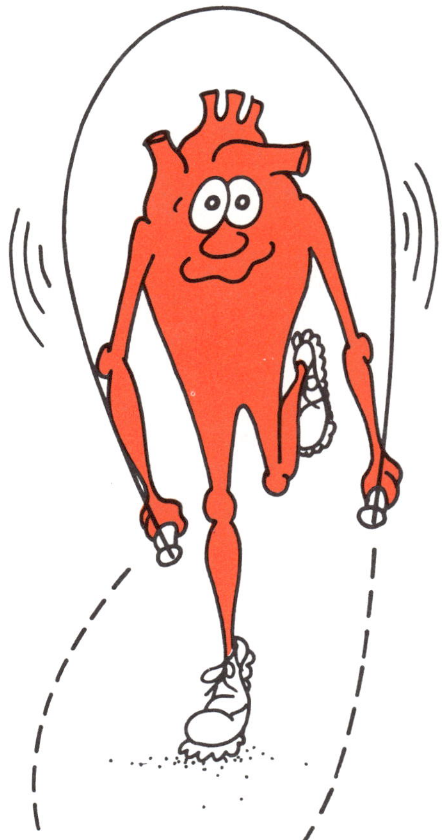

Work Out

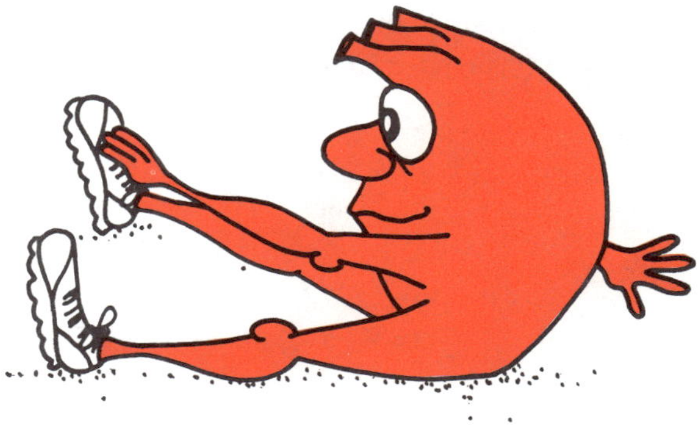

Cool Down

Once your doctor has approved a type and amount of exercise for you, here are some tips to help you stick to it:

1. **Start off slowly.** Add vigor when you have begun to build up some strength. This may take a few weeks or months. Pay attention to how your muscles and body feel. You will soon know when it's time to slow down or speed up during exercise.

2. **Regular exercise** means either:

- every other day
- 3 or 4 times a week
- 2 days on and 1 day off

Doing it this way gives the muscles time to refuel for the next workout. You work the body, then let it rest. Not only do the above routines help prevent injuries, the pace keeps your interest up. Do not go at exercise like a loose train and then take 2 or 3 weeks off to recover. This is not safe, and injuries are common.

3. **Do something you enjoy.** You simply won't keep doing an exercise if you don't like it. This is why walking is so popular. It's easy and can be done indoors or outside. Good shoes and comfortable clothes are the only expense for walking.

4. **Choose an exercise partner** if you need an extra push. A friend, dog or video exercise program can help you plan and stick to an exercise routine.

Not smoking

If you don't already know what smoking can do to your health, here are some of the risks that smokers face:

- more heart disease and heart attacks
- more lung disease and lung cancer
- more fatty buildup in the arteries
- poor blood flow

If you have high blood pressure and are also a smoker, your risks for heart and lung disease are doubled. So think about it, and try anything to quit smoking.

Most towns now have stop-smoking clinics to help you. Your own hospital is a good place to call about such a group.

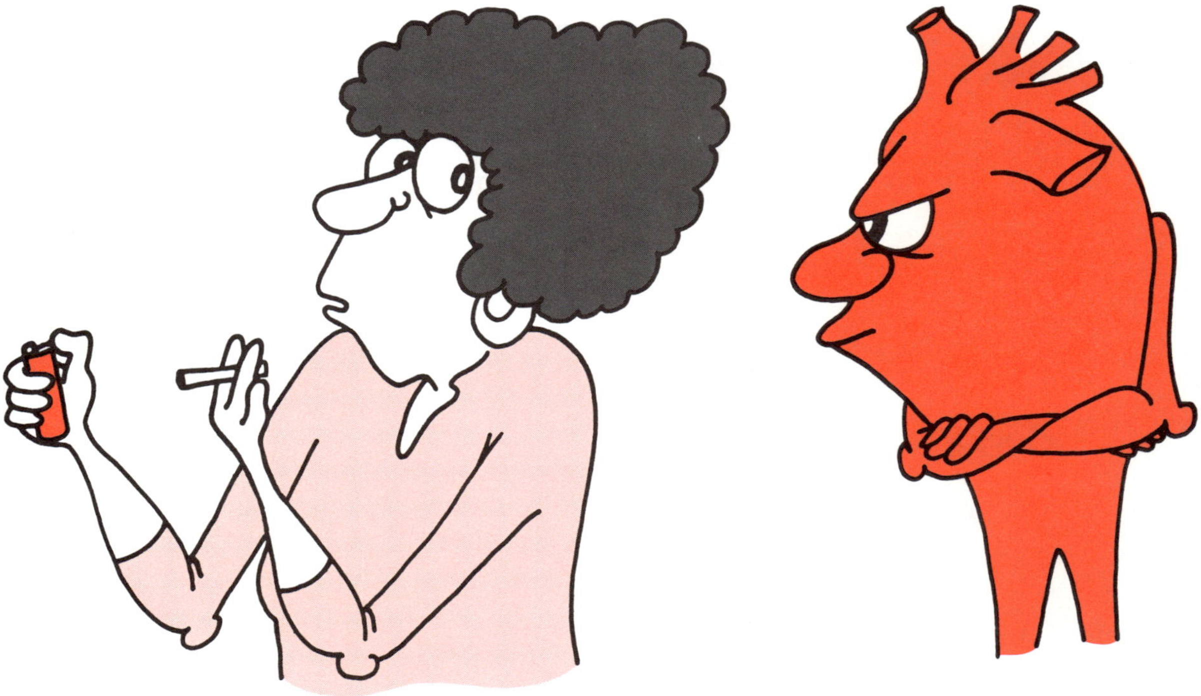

Taking your own blood pressure

Your doctor may ask that you take your blood pressure at home. If so, you should know that:

- blood pressure is often low when you have been asleep
- blood pressure goes up as you wake up and become more active
- sudden stress or pain can cause blood pressure to rise in a few seconds

When you take your own blood pressure, take it at about the same time each day and in the same surroundings.

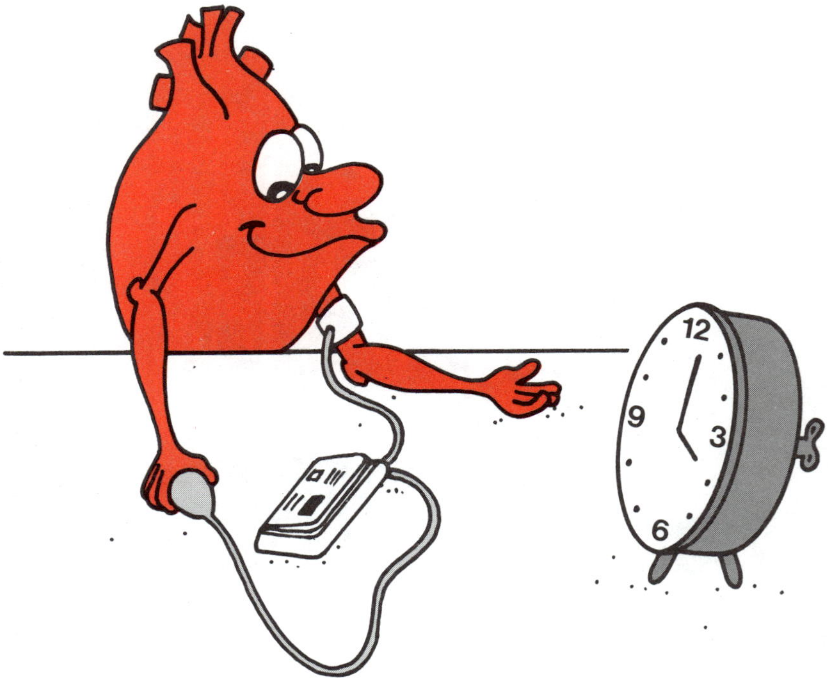

The device used to take your blood pressure is called a sphygmomanometer. The 3 types you can buy are listed on these next pages.

Types of equipment

Mercury

This is the blood pressure device most often seen in a doctor's office. It is the most accurate since less can go wrong with it. It is not likely you would buy one of these for your home, but it would be a good idea to check out the one you buy with the one in your doctor's office. Then you will know if your home device is giving you a true reading.

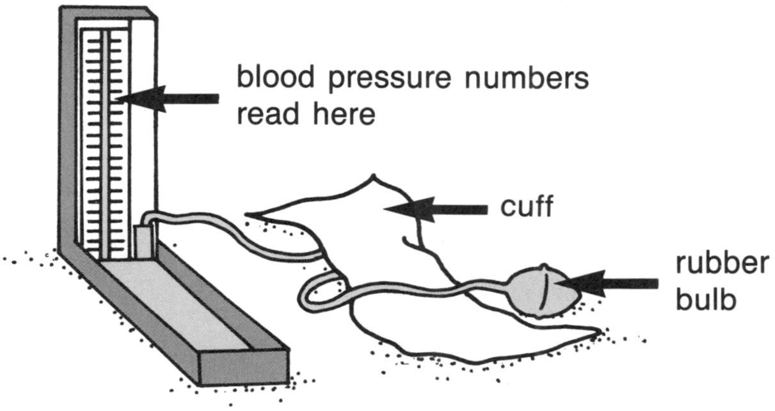

Aneroid (no liquid)

This device is more delicate than the mercury-type. If you buy one of these, check it out with the device your doctor uses. Do this about every 6 months.

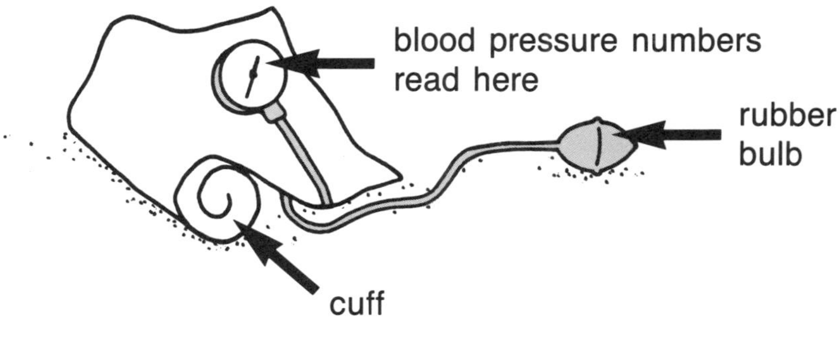

Digital (computer numbers)

The most popular device today is a digital blood pressure device. These are not too costly, and blood pressure is easy to read in the numbers flashed on a small screen. Some also have a paper printout (like on a calculator) that gives you your blood pressure reading. As with the aneroid, check a digital device with your doctor's to make sure it is accurate.

Important tips on digital sphygmomanometers:

1. All digital blood pressure equipment comes with instructions. Read them carefully before starting to take a blood pressure.

2. Store the blood pressure device at room temperature. Extreme heat or cold can cause it to give wrong readings.

3. Home gauges may become inaccurate. Take yours with you to your doctor, and check it by his or her blood pressure device.

4. The height at which you hold your arm can affect the blood pressure reading. Keep the arm around which you wrap the blood pressure cuff at about heart level. Do this by propping the arm up on a table, sofa edge, etc.

Technique

Read through these steps one or more times before starting.

1. Sit in a quiet place near a table where you can place your arm and equipment comfortably.

2. Wrap the blood pressure cuff around your bare arm (not over your clothes) an inch above the elbow. The cuff should fit snugly but with enough room so that one finger can be slipped under the cuff. Wrap the cuff evenly.

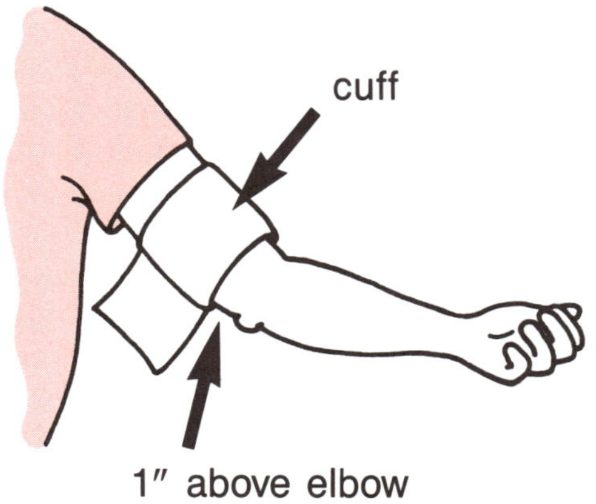

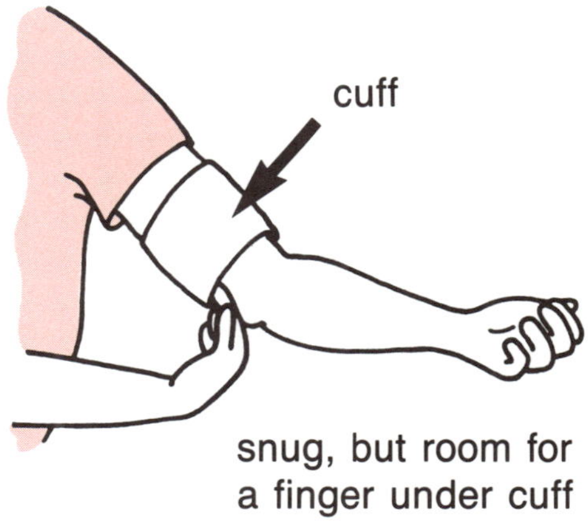

3. Rest your elbow and lower arm on the table so that the upper arm is level with the heart. Stay still.

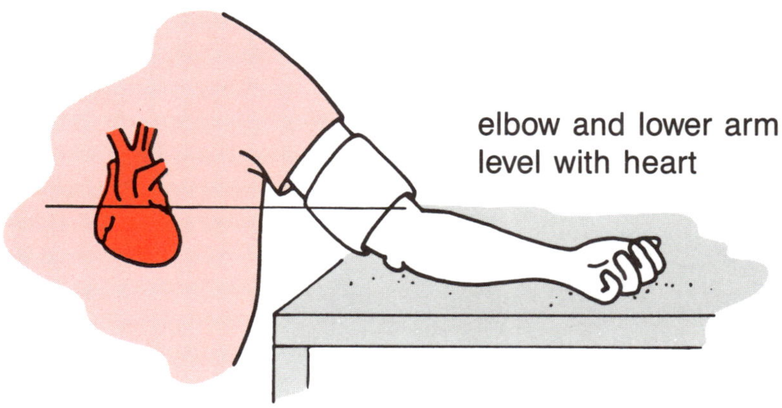

4. Turn the power on.

5. Squeeze the rubber bulb and inflate the cuff.* Inflate the cuff about 30-40 mmHg above the estimated systolic pressure. (This is the level of blood pressure that causes the radial pulse to disappear when the cuff is pumped up.)

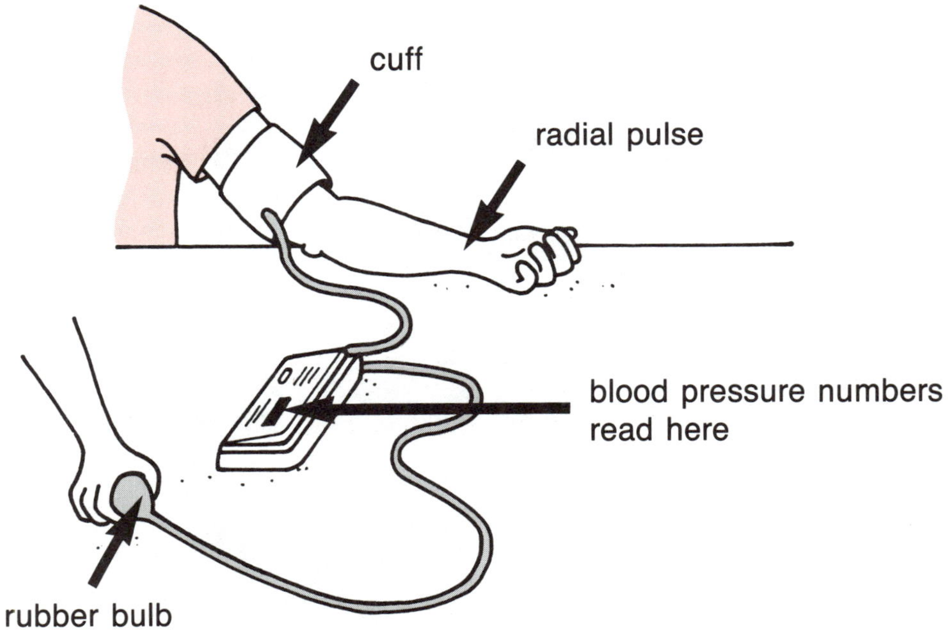

6. After you stop inflating, the automatic exhaust mechanism will slowly reduce the cuff pressure. The machine will display your systolic and diastolic pressures on the screen.

7. Press the exhaust button to release all of the air from the cuff.

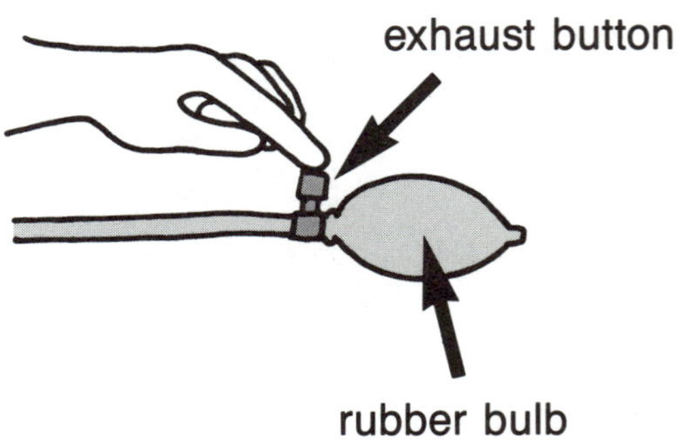

8. Turn power off.

*Some cuffs don't have a rubber bulb and inflate automatically with the push of a button.

Keep these in mind when taking your blood pressure:

Taking your blood pressure over clothes or rolling a shirt or jacket up over the upper arm, can cause false or high readings.

Many machines offer only one size of cuff. But cuffs must be large enough to get a true reading. Measure the distance around the middle of your upper arm. If it is more than about 13 inches, you will need a large rather than a standard size cuff. If the standard size cuff is used on a person with large arms, the blood pressure reading may be falsely high.

If the arm being used for taking your blood pressure is higher than the heart, the pressure may show up as lower than the true value. If the arm is lower than the heart, the reading may show higher than the true value.

This equipment should be stored with care. Remove the batteries before storing the machine. Make sure tubing is not twisted when stored. Store your equipment away from heat and dust. Check rubber tubing for cracks or leaks.

Some final words

You now know what treatment of high blood pressure includes. You also know how to take your own blood pressure if needed. As you bring your blood pressure down, you and your doctor are partners. For this to work, you must stay in touch with your doctor. He or she needs to know your progress and change treatment when needed. Don't wait until a heart attack, stroke, kidney or eye complication proves to you that high blood pressure is serious. It is. Learn to eat right, keep a trim weight, take medications as prescribed, relax, stop smoking and exercise regularly. These will increase your chances for a full, healthy life. Get in control, and stay there. This book can help you get started.

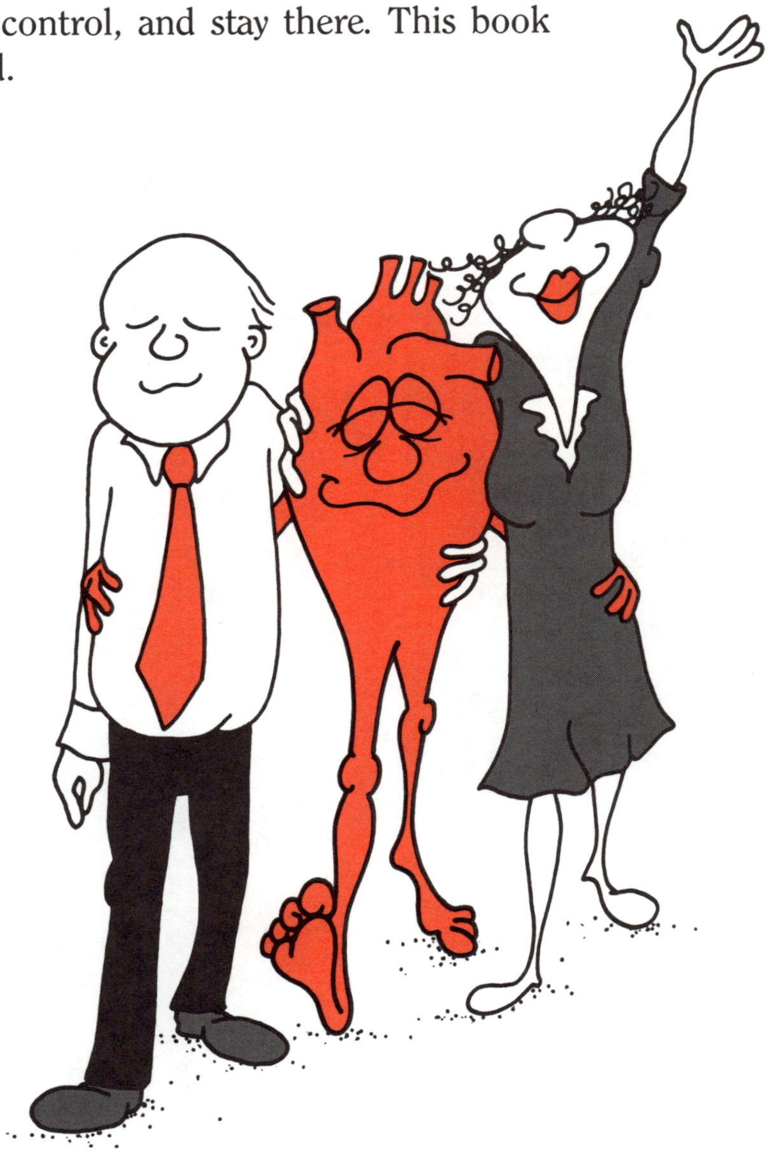

Stay in Control!